MW01101617

Strange Encounters
With Carl Auer

. . . .

Strange Encounters With Carl Auer

. . . .

Edited by Gunthard Weber and Fritz B. Simon

W. W. NORTON & COMPANY

NEW YORK • • • LONDON

Printed in the United States of America.

First Edition

Library of Congress Cataloging-in-Publication Data

Carl Auer, English.
   Strange encounters with Carl Auer / Gunthard Weber and Fritz
B. Simon.
      p.   cm.
   Translation of : Carl Auer.
   ISBN 0-393-03068-7 : $19.95
   I. Weber, Gunthard. II. Simon, Fritz B. III. Title.
PT2660.A1C3713 1991   833'.914—dc20   91–24730

W. W. Norton & Company, Inc., 500 Fifth Avenue, New York, N.Y. 10110
W. W. Norton & Company, Ltd., 10 Coptic Street, London WC1 1PU

1 2 3 4 5 6 7 8 9 0

Table of Contents

How to Five
Editors' Preface

Probably no other personality of our time has divided opinion so sharply as Carl Auer. It is indeed possible to split up the human species into those who love and revere him and those who don't. And this second group can in its turn be divided into those who would love and revere him if they knew he existed and those who probably, or quite definitely, wouldn't. Although Carl Auer has always been a declared enemy of the appalling oversimplification that such binary oppositions represent, he in fact signals his agreement in this particular instance when he remarks: "I have always loved and revered the second group."

We thus had no occasion to be surprised by the difficulties we encountered in coming within hailing distance of the Carl Auer phenomenon. He had after all spent all his life combating the idealization of personalities in whatever form and crusading with equal acrimony against the personalization of ideas. And to say that we received any kind of cooperation or encouragement from him in our intention of publishing a book on the man and his ideas (if it is indeed possible to separate the two) would be a wilful misrepresentation of the facts. We wanted him to tell us everything, he didn´t want to tell us anything. Only very reluctantly did he finally agree to withdraw a court order prohibiting any kind of homage to, or appreciation of, his merits and achievements. Unpredictable as ever, he made his ultimate acquiescence conditional upon having the establishment publishing the *festschrift* in honor of his 90th birthday named after him. If this ultimatum was designed to deflect us from our purpose, then it failed to achieve the desired result, as the present volume attests. Instead, Carl Auer has once again been responsible for a new departure. Alongside all his other pioneering ventures, he has now become the initiator of a new publishing press bearing his name (whether posterity will reckon this among his achievements is arguable given the glut of printed matter on the market and the consequent disorientation of the potential reader).

If we decided to persevere in our intention of publishing a volume devoted to Carl Auer, then it is largely because of his outstanding significance for our own personal development and that of many others as well. In critical situations encountered in our private and professional lives we knew that Carl Auer was there to proffer advice and assistance. Even if he usually appeared somewhat absent on such occasions, it was his way of thinking and feeling, sometimes the suspicion of unashamedly tasteless humor and invariably the creative spark he communicated that showed us the way out of some apparent impasse, opened up new avenues or inspired us to feats of visionary, innovative thinking accompanied by loud cries of "eureka!". In short, our debt to Carl Auer is immense, he has been our guiding light.

Since the publication of his *magnum opus* "Between Fear and Sex", his influence on the development of western culture and academic and scientific endeavor has been palpable indeed. Carl Auer has done as much to query and shake the very foundations of western thought as he has to confirm its significance and extend its frontiers. His publications, and even more so his own life, have been devoted to revealing the absurdity of distinctions hitherto taken for granted, such as those between raw and cooked, man and woman, sensory and extra-sensory, intellect and emotion, body and soul, German and English, abstract and concrete, future and time, right and space, all of them polarizations which he has passionately and radically shown up for the fictions they are.

His has been a life full of contradictions. At home in many languages, Auer has always rebelled against the restrictions imposed by dictionaries and grammar books, exploring with inimitable gusto the limitless semantic freedoms afforded by a multilingual approach to meaning and thought. A major thinker, he began at the tender age of 14 to preoccupy himself with all conceivable and apperceptible phenomena of *Geist*, more specifically with the interrelations that exist between the various meanings of that word, Geist as mind, spirit and spectre. Was this, as some historians have claimed, the birth of self-referentiality? Or are these enthusiastic, albeit occasionally no more than spirited, reports of his sensory and extra-sensory experiences traceable to the inspiriting influence of alcohol? What relation exists between body and *Geist* (in all its forms)? Is there in fact such a relation at all?

This of course is a question that we as editors of this volume have been constantly preoccupied with. The spirit of Carl Auer is all-pervasive and yet Auer himself is always on the verge of disappearing like a spirit in the mists of impenetrable contradiction. As we felt incapable of broaching the question of the truth about Auer on our own, we elected to make a virtue of necessity and request prominent personalities who have encountered Auer to give an impression of their experiences with him. We should like to express our gratitude for the promptness with which they acceded to this request. The result is a mosaic, a coruscating, multi-faceted compendium of glimpses and vignettes, made up of sketches, letters and anecdotes all reflecting Auer´s major interests and concerns, a collection of accounts covering the whole gamut of feelings between fear and sex, full of passion and adventure, intellectuality and worldly wisdom, banality and genius, unconventionality and conformity, revealing Auer as a unique blend of the subversive and the survivor.

As Auer himself put it quite recently: "True greatness reveals itself in the acceptance of one´s own mediocrity!" It was on the basis of this conviction that he insisted that he was one of the greatest figures of his age. He has always been extremely reticent on the point, however, for, as he has often said, if there is one thing he is proud of it is his humility.

Auer's own response to the existential question that he poses in his major work ("What comes between fear and sex[1]?") finds him crossing the boundaries of language again. His answer is: "fünf!" (="five").

Where a more conventional mind would be tempted to concentrate on the dark animal impulses of human nature, Auer suddenly brings in the quantitative, precisely mathematical element. Here we have the quintessential Auer, the wanderer between psychoanalysis and mathematics. It is thus that he shakes us out of the deceptive security of a complacent, impermeable, cut-and-dried system of blind self-satisfied specialism. He forces us to cross boundaries and face up to contradictions.

9

For this reason we have refrained from imposing a spurious consistency on the apparent logical or temporal contradictions that obtain between some of the reports and interpretations of the authors assembled here. All we have done is to compile the (admittedly incomplete) data on Auer in the form of a table of facts and figures. But it may well have been the deeper motive behind Auer's signal lack of cooperation to force the reader to draw his own conclusions. Our Auer is not everybody's Auer. His true nature was, is and will perhaps remain an enigma, spectral, impalpable.

For all its apparent obviousness, his insistence that five comes between fear (four) and sex (six) is no real aid to comprehension. Does this really represent the synthesis (in Hegel's sense) of the conflict between quantity and quality? This would only be the case if we knew what "5" really means for Auer. What does fiving imply for him, how does one actually go about it? This is a topic which we may safely predict, will be preoccupying critics and academics throughout the decades to come. Carl Auer's own answer to the question of "how to five" was in many ways typical: "Just five in at the deep end!"

Heidelberg, summer 1990
Fritz B. Simon and Gunthard Weber

---

[1] *vier* (pronounced as "fear") and *sechs* (pronounced "sex") in German are the words for "four" and "six" respectively.

Acknowledgements

All those persons who have time and again encouraged and energetically supported us in daring this first attempt at an estimation of Carl Auer deserve our special thanks. The constant flow of unexpected information made the typing and desk-top-publishing tasks of Ms. Syska and Ms. Fisher especially wearisome; their contribution deserves our thanks as well. Sally and Bernd Hofmeister and Andrew Jenkins helped some of the texts to "speak two languages." Neither do we want to leave unmentioned all those souls whose colorful contributions we could not include for the sole reason that these accounts did not stand up to rigorous academic investigation. This was the case, for example, with a resident of a home for the aged in the north of Baden, S. C. Hertz, who used to play in a sandbox with Carl Auer, as well as a Carl-Auer-infatuated woman who was vacationing in Greece.

Heidelberg, October, 1990
The Editors

Inner Formation
Instead of Information

Watersheds of Understanding
Ernst von Glasersfeld

> The droplet frosting cleaves the mountains' night,
> Thus wisdom's word the world refashions quite.
> Pang-Chi-Yu (17th century)[1]

The news that Carl Auer will be celebrating his ninetieth birthday this autumn came as a considerable shock. For some fifty years now he has played the role of an inadvertent but extremely influential mentor to me. I say inadvertent because he is presumably oblivious of any kind of relationship between us, influential because, looking back, I see that my encounters with him, although not initially understood as such, were encounters of a kind that mark one for life.

My first reaction to the invitation to contribute to this *festschrift* was the chastening reflection that, as both of us are now well-stricken in years, it becomes less and less likely as time passes that the future will hold any further "chance" encounters with this unique personality. This was soon compounded with the paralyzing diffidence that befalls one upon being actually confronted, for the first time, with an all but mythical figure one has hitherto revered from a safe distance. So this is probably the last opportunity I shall have of giving anything like an unself-conscious account of the circumstances in which contact with Carl Auer has been the source of entirely novel insights.

I

The first encounter, though I failed to recognize it as such, took place in impenetrable fog. For two years it was to remain as unforgettable as it was incomprehensible. When I was a student in the mid-1930s, I took every available opportunity to go on skiing expeditions in the glacier regions of the Austrian Alps. On such excursions it is by no means unusual for the weather to play tricks on one, and thus it was that, in the course of an ascent to one of those Alpine shelter huts that one has to cross the glaciers to get to, Irene, my companion at that time, and I found ourselves suddenly shrouded in fog. Only someone who knows the mountains can have so much as an inkling of what fog at that altitude can do. It creates a world in which all visible distinctions and outlines are lost, one can literally see no further than the end of one's skis. The driving snow forms a completely uniform expanse of whiteness in which the sky above and the earth beneath are as one and there is no discernible horizon or any other landmark from which to take one's bearings. The situation is comparable to that of those unfortunate animals that experimental psychologists observe to see how they react when a translucent sphere similar to a giant ping-pong ball is tied around their heads, allowing the passage of light but not the usual perception of contours, let alone "objects."

I made my way forward with small, regular steps, my sole concern being to proceed in as straight a line as possible. Suddenly, only a few yards in front of me a shadow emerged from the white, swirling, broth-like element around me, a man on skis, coming in our direction. His sudden appearance was so startling that we almost collided.

"Noli tangere circulos meos," he called cheerily and without coming to a halt. Like ourselves he had the hood of his ski parka well down over his eyes and was wearing snow-goggles. No face was discernible. He negotiated the obstacle we represented with a skating step before continuing his descent in the tracks we had left and seemed to hesitate for an instant and then called over his shoulder: "As long as we come full circle we have not lost our way!" The next moment he was swallowed up by the mist in the direction we had come from.

Astonishment had taken our breath away. As I was occupied in taking out two apples from my rucksack, we experienced one of those moments which make one suddenly forget the rigors of such an ascent. In a blinding flash of sunlight the white void around us was suddenly riven, and before we could bite into our apples the fog miraculously lifted and disappeared. The broad expanse of the glacier lay before us, the peaks reared like monuments of ice that we could reach out and touch, the sky arched like a vault of deep blue above us.

It was then that we saw the broad circle, as yet hardly snowed over, that the stranger had left in the expanse of virgin snow all around, a circle to which our own tracks stood as an accurate tangent. He had obviously been going around in that circle for some time as there was no vestige of any track that might have shown how he got there.

But the most astounding thing of all was yet to come. We discovered it as we were about to resume the ascent. With his skiing-pole he had written something in the snow, in large letters along the circumference of the circle. I almost fell over myself in my eagerness to decipher what I was convinced would be an important message. And there, still legible, stood the words: "From night to night, a ladder from nowhere to nought."

When we finally resumed our course we repeated to ourselves those enticingly arcane words until they merged into the very rhythms of our motion. Although we had no notion of their profounder significance, they became as it were the refrain of our ascents and the brief span of our togetherness.

II

Almost exactly two years later, Hitler had just marched into Austria, I was passing through Zurich. I decided to phone Irene. I had not seen her for some time but there had been a cordial, if occasional, change of letters.

"Hallo," she said and then, after recovering from her initial suprise, "I know you've been worried about me, but there's no need now"; then, after a slight hesitation, "As long as we come full circle, we have not lost our way: I'm getting married next week."

I was touched and gladdened by this news, wished her much joy and repaired to the dentist's where I had contrived to get myself an appointment at short notice. Listlessly thumbing my way through one of the so-called "radical" literary journals of the time in the waiting-room, I suddenly came upon the very same words we had stumbled across in the mountain snows two years before.

My heart began to thump in a most unruly manner. Here were those very words, as part of a poem quoted in the course of a book-review. The relevant section read as follows:

The young scientist Carl Auer who relinquished his research post in Austria a year before the anschluss in order to devote himself to studies of a private nature in Hintertüpfli near Appenzell has published a volume of delightful parodies.

Instead of the usual analysis we have chosen to reproduce one of these confections here, entitled by Auer, "Sonnet to Prometheus, after R. M. Rilke":

> Tethered and blind,
> with futile tools
> fools grope to find
> a soothing truth in rules.
>
> No one attains a rhyme
> to weave a world together,
> to last forever
> against the blast of time.
>
> From night to night
> the ladder grows.
> Thought upon thought
>
> into the darkness reason throws,
> from nowhere to nought,
> but a transient spark of light.[2]

I tore the page out of the magazine and took it away with me, of course with the intention of looking for the book. I was convinced that this Carl Auer and the man in the fog were one and the same person. The following evening, however, in the third-class compartment of a crowded train to Paris, I suddenly started having doubts. The man in the fog might have been a friend of Carl Auer's, who, upon being shown the budding poet's efforts had said with the typical heartlessness of youth: "My dear Carl, this is no good at all. You can pass it off as a Rilke parody if you like, but you can't publish it as a poem of your own."

III

Anyone who ever travelled overnight by train in those years will remember that reading was anything but easy. Even the long-distance trains had to economize on electricity and the light from the grimy light-bulbs in the third class was murky indeed. Soon after we left Zurich my fellow passengers lapsed into deep slumber. My thoughts revolved around the man in the fog and his poem. In order to reread it I had to hunch myself forward and hold the crumpled page up before my eyes. The fourth or fifth time I did this, I noticed that the man next to me was awake. "Carl is a wizard!" he said, in a hoarse whisper addressed more to himself than to anyone else. Without waiting for any affirmation on my part he carried on in broad Swiss dialect, manifestly at pains not to awaken any of the sleepers. Not once did he raise his voice, and yet he evinced an enthusiasm that I had never encountered before from the inhabitants of that region on any subject. Although I had difficulty understanding his dialect after all those years, I was still able to glean from this whispered outburst details that I could hardly have learned from any other source.

The first thing I was told was that my fellow-traveller was a member of the Cantonal Council of Appenzell and that this Council had just decided to make Professor Auer a freeman of the canton. "Because he's so good at writing parodies?" I asked, amazed. (Having spent much of my youth in Switzerland I knew by experience how unlikely it was that that country's smallest canton should feel moved to make literary gestures of such a nature.) My neighbor ignored the question altogether and resumed his whispered monologue. I should probably have shared his excitement if I had known what heroic deed it was that had prompted Appenzell to give Carl Auer a reward beyond the wildest dreams of a Central European refugee in those years. But it was only when my neighbor started getting his things together to leave the train in Bern that I had the chance to ask what it was that he had done.

For the first time since we had left Zurich he turned to me, his face the epitome of incredulity. "You mean you don't know? You've not heard?" While maneuvering his luggage down from the rack he said something of which it was only the very last word that caused me no problems of interpretation. That word was "castrated." Then my friend from Appenzell squeezed his way out of the compartment and disappeared.

A dozen other questions were clamouring for an answer in my head. One of them was, of course, whether Professor Auer was a skier. I was tempted to get out, there and then, in order to find out more about Carl Auer. But wiser councils prevailed; I had more important worries on my mind.

As I continued my journey I did my best to arrive at a clearer understanding of what I had heard and to find some plausible explanation. It appeared that the production of Appenzell's famous cheese had been all but brought to a standstill by the appearance of a hitherto unknown insect. I cannot say whether it was an insect of the winged variety, whether it was of a biting or stinging persuasion, as the only definition they had for it in Appenzell was "devil-mite." The source of the mortal fear that this apocalyptic insect had instilled in them was that it influenced either the cows or the milk or the cheese-making process in such a way that the product had no longer so much as a vestige of the flavor that had made it world-famous. The implications for the economic survival of the area, perhaps even for the whole canton, were of course catastrophic. The crisis had reached its climax when Professor Auer arrived in the neighborhood and rented rooms there. Of course he was soon apprised of the emergency and (this is at least my own possibly too prosaic view) as he probably knew how difficult it was to obtain an unlimited residence permit for Switzerland, the first thing he turned his attention to, when he had set up a small laboratory in his garret, was the Appenzell Cheese Problem.

As so often happened, Carl Auer was successful. A few weeks later he informed the postmaster (possibly the only native that he had managed to exchange a few words with in the first few months of his stay) that he thought he might be able to help.

My fellow-traveller's narration became so confused at this point that I can venture no more than a vague hypothesis about the nature of the miracle wrought by Carl Auer. Apparently he succeeded in isolating one of those hitherto unknown sex-related substances that the nervous system of certain insects is one hundred percent responsive to, and not only that but also to produce that substance independently. Thereupon - and this is perhaps an even more astonishing achievement - he managed to convince the elders of the community of the plausibility of his plan. It seems as if in the course of that winter vast amounts of that mysterious substance were in fact produced in the giant cheese vats of the dairies. Then - and if I know Carl Auer at all this will have appealed particularly strongly to his predilection for irony - the substance was taken out in the course of those local spring festivities that are a remnant of pre-Christian fertility rites and pasted over the tree-trunks of the entire vicinity by every single member of the local population. No sooner were the odious insects hatched than the males flocked to the irresistible bait, there to squander their entire reproductive potential - or as my informant put it, they were "castrated." (Anyone familiar with our author may be tempted to interpret this episode as the source of Auer's later highly controversial suggestions with regard to the problem of overpopulation.)

Although I am convinced that, in essentials at least, the information given to me by the stranger on the train was not mere invention, my hypothetical interpretation is of course a daring one, and certainly requires further substantiation, particularly as my excitable friend constantly compared Professor Auer to "Doktor Faustus" and also used the terms "witches' broth" and "black magic." On the other hand, what I later read concerning Carl Auer's work in such a wide range of different branches did go some way towards substantiating my version. One of the essential principles postulated by that great scholar is that effective change can only be achieved via approaches that the organism in question is already familiar with. It was thus to be expected that such an unprejudiced and clear-headed thinker as Carl Auer would attack organisms where they are most familiar, i. e. in their sexuality.

In the turmoil of the months that followed, spent largely in search of a place where I would be allowed to stay even though I could not work miracles, I put the whole affair completely out of my mind.

IV

The next indirect encounter was of a different kind, but no less astonishing. About five years after the events in Switzerland, I was in Dublin with my young wife. James Joyce's last work *Finnegan's Wake* had just come out. As great admirers of Joyce we bought the book immediately and tried to read it, both separately and jointly. One morning as I was in the bathroom shaving, my wife called out: "What are . . ."and then an incomprehensible word. I wiped my face, went to the bed and read the passage my wife indicated. The passage was as follows:

In newrotic ages the pterobly dactile carlosaurian engentians earnest machinations on the vicotorious march of skientific progress to the iambatistan rhythm of Himmelayan pistemologies.[3]

The allusion to Giambattista Vico was obvious. A reading of the first page of the book in the company of friends had already brought us up against the Italian philosopher. Nor was Ernst Mach difficult to detect. But I had to reduce the passage to its constituent syllables before I became aware of the presence of Carl Auer. Not, of course, that one could be absolutely sure. The name Carlo is not so rare and there was nothing about the link with the saurians to make certain identification any easier. But "ski" and "gentian" were a patent reference to the mountains.

Suddenly I realized that I had never told my wife of my pre-war encounters with Carl Auer. When I had made good this omission as best I could, she said: "Carl Auer, Carl Auer, I think I once came across an article of his in the library. I remember thinking that the title sounded like Wagner, 'The Ring of Neuro-Linkages' or something like that."

We unearthed the journal in the library and the article was indeed entitled "The Ring of Neuro-Linkages: Inner Formation instead of Information."[4] Condensed in the space of two pages, we found here not only the concept of the closed system but the whole range of unnerving consequences that this idea had for biology as well as cognitive development and epistemology. To be honest, we understood very little of what he was saying. The neurobiological examples he quoted required specialized knowledge that we were not even remotely possessed of. But there was one passage that I found acutely gratifying. Unfortunately I have since mislaid the article but the message of the passage in question has remained inscribed indelibly on my mind.

In a section with the knee-weakeningly allusive sub-heading "The Biological *Noli Tangere*," Auer set out to demonstrate that in the last resort living beings had only one aim and that was the preservation of their inner harmony. In the course of time what they feel to be constituent of that harmony may change. But if it changes in such a way to make it harder to preserve and to require even greater sacrifices, then there is going to be trouble. Once such a risky course has been embarked upon then even a slight shift in environmental conditions can trigger a disaster. The fate of the dinosaurs, whose weight, strength and hence cell proliferation developed at the expense of everything else was, Auer said, a grim warning to avoid any one-sided development. (A footnote referred to a more detailed discussion of this point by the author elsewhere.[5])

This then was the link-up with the "circles" that we must not break, with the dinosaurs, and finally with the manic fear of unambiguity that makes *Finnegans Wake* all but unreadable. There was now no doubt that the man in the fog was Carl Auer, here delineated clearly as an unflinchingly innovative thinker and the founder of a pioneering philosophical approach.

In addition, the article contained a multitude of terms which were extremely unfamiliar in those days, such as "mono-autonomy," "co-phenomenal," "self-concatenation" which must have taken root in my unconscious only to emerge at a later date in my own work. This, of course, must not be taken to mean that I understood them in the sense that Carl Auer was using them, only that (as with so many others) time and my own experience finally made it possible for me to invest them with some kind of sense.

V

Then came World-War II and the postwar years, a long period in which one had little inclination to reminisce about past experiences. It must have been when I was working in Milan around 1950 that a colleague of mine showed me the announcement of a lecture by a visiting professor. The Italian title intrigued me: *La problematica delle soluzione.* Preoccupied as I was day and night with translation, I automatically asked myself whether this meant the problem of finding solutions or the problems that solutions bring with them.

It was then that I read the name Carlo Auer. And in my mind's eye I saw an unrecognizable and yet not unfamiliar figure coming towards me out of the fog, like all those years before, on the glacier.

As far as lectures were concerned I had already gathered some considerable experience. Without actually admitting it to myself I tended to divide them up into two groups, those (rare) occasions on which one does one's best to follow what the speaker is saying and all those others, where the main problem is to conceal both from one's colleagues and the speaker, that one has lapsed into profound torpor. No sooner had Carl Auer mounted the platform that I knew that this was going to be a different experience altogether.

Of course, it would be absurd to suggest that I recognized him. I had only seen him in snow-goggles and a hood covering the rest of his face. But the very way he scaled the platform immediately marked him out as a mountaineer. He grasped the edge of the lectern with both hands as if he were about to thrust himself downhill on a pair of skis. With head bent and shoulders slightly raised, the classic posture one might say, he began his remarks in fluent, indeed excellent Italian and spoke without interval, sometimes more slowly but never faltering. His whole body was attuned to the rhythms of his speech, just as a skillful skier will unconsciously match his every movement to the rises and hollows of the ground he is negotiating. I was fascinated, no less by the physical dynamism of the man than by what he actually had to say.

Other contributors to this *festschrift* are undoubtedly more competent than I to situate the work of Carl Auer in the history of Western thought. I took it to be the central idea of his lecture in Milan that, necessary as it may be to look for the solution to a problem in one direction or another, it invariably has embarassing not to say devastating consequences to indulge in the fond belief that the solution we find is the *right* one and hence the only possible one.

At the end of his lecture, Carl Auer summed up the essence of his philosophy in a play on words that casts far more light on his true nature than I ever could. And it is with this profound pun that I shall close my account of these quasi-encounters with the great man, whom I have not in fact ever seen again.

Even before the applause had ebbed away, people started thronging the platform from all corners of the room. I followed suit, but was unable to get anywhere near the speaker. A group of self-important "colleagues" monopolized him so successfully that the less impertinent questioners finally turned away in disappointment. But then a German voice bellowed from some distance back: "Herr Professor, what is your opinion of Ernst Mach?" Carl Auer, who thus far had inclined a patient, albeit not tremendously enthusiastic ear to the questions of those beleaguering him, suddenly drew himself up to his full height, cast an irresistibly satirical glance at the earnest, bespectacled gentleman who had asked the question and then gave his answer, not only to the inquirer but to the whole world: "I owe a great deal to Ernst Mach but I think I match Ernst as far as sensational analysis is concerned!" With that he bowed and sailed out of the hall with consummate elegance.

Envoy

How often does a man of words, be he scientist or poet, look down at the sentence he has just written and say: Where did I get that from? Is it really my own idea?

In recent years doubts of this nature have been assailing me more and more frequently. And summoning up these memories of events that I have only inadequately recounted here has all but confirmed my suspicions. As I see it, it is Carl Auer - the only contemporary whom the term "Renaissance Man" really seems to fit - who in fact said more or less everything that I have laboriously fumbled together myself. Presumably that should be a source of mortification to me. But it isn´t. The myriad echoes that I now think I can discern in my work give me a deeper satisfaction. Those insights of Carl Auer's that were most influential for me now appear so important for the salvation of our ailing world that the question of who expressed or repeated them when and where is of small moment. And quite aside from that, Carl Auer is probably the last person who would claim author's rights.

Hence I look forward to this birthday celebration and the first "real" encounter with my inadvertent mentor with an easy conscience and more than pleasurable anticipation.

Notes

[1]Klabund, *Chinesische Gedichte*. Zürich: Phaidon, 1954, p. 14.

[2]*Die gelbe Spinne*, März 1937, Jahrgang 3, Nr. 1, p. 12.

[3] James Joyce, *Finnegan's Wake*. London: Faber & Faber, 1939, p. 19 (passage later deleted by the author).

[4]Carl Auer, "The Ring of Neuro-Linkages: Inner Formation Instead of Information," *Nature*, 1943, 79, pp. 273-275.

[5]Carl Auer, "Die Versponnenheit der Saurier," *Neue Naturwissenschaft*, 1939, 13, p. 79-87.

You Cannot Cross
a River Once

Tell Me Carl, Where Do I Exist?

Karl Tomm

The wood was burning feverishly as I threw in another log and quickly closed the door. The stove was hot, really hot! But it needed to be . It was another one of those cold winter nights in the Canadian Rockies - it must have been at least 30 degrees below zero! Maybe even 35! And it was very dark outside.The snow-capped mountains and the frozen lake were barely visible in the twinkling starlight.

Fortunately, the little stove threw a lot of heat. The young salesman said it would, and I was glad that he was right. Despite the cold, it was able to keep the whole cabin warm. He said the stove had been built in New Zealand and was designed for efficiency. It burned not only the wood but also the gases released from the wood before they went up the chimney. The idea was intriguing at the time, but actually seeing it happen was even more so. Through the big glass window at the front of the stove, I could see the flames dancing with the gases right there in front of me. It was an exquisite and fascinating sight!

I leaned back into the large soft cushions on the floor as I watched the fire burn. The sound of the crackling blaze and the smell of hot charred wood added to the warmth and comfort in the cabin as I imagined the contrasting cold outside. It was a wonderful place to relax and reflect. I could spend hours in the cabin simply staring into the hypnotic dance of undulating flames as they were glowing in the dark.

On this particular occasion, I found myself in a deep conversation with a delightful old man. He was the kind of person one often imagines when thinking about the author of a great philosophical work - thoughtful, wise, and dignified. I think his name was Carl von Auer but I can't be sure. It is mainly the conversation itself that I recall. Just how it happened that we came to be together at the cabin that night remains a mystery. Sometimes I even wonder if it didn't all take place in my imagination and if the conversation I had wasn't really with myself! Perhaps I slipped into a trance as I was watching the mesmerizing fire. The dancing flames triggered a personal philosophical question that had been haunting me for some time:

"Carl, how can I know that I, Karl, am anything more than a dynamic swirl of pure process like those flames?"

He was resting casually on the floor about a meter to my left. With his head and shoulders propped up on a large red pillow, he was also gazing into the blazing fire. "What a delightful thought!" he said. "I am very impressed with your empathy and humility today!"

"Now just hang on here! I didn't say there was nothing more to me than a flame! I asked an honest question and you side-stepped it." I thought that he had deliberately misunderstood and admit I felt a tinge of annoyance.

"O.K., O.K.," he said calmly. "It's just that it sounded like such a refreshingly humble way to think of oneself in this age of arrogance."

"Are you implying that it would be arrogant of me to say that as a human being I am more than a dancing flame?"

"No, not necessarily. It depends on the manner and context in which you make the claim."

"Well, I'm thinking of myself as a living organism, and as a human being that *knows* that he is alive. I don't think we can say that of the flame."

"O.K., I could agree with you on that. . . . So what's your question?"

"Well, when I wonder what I am, I look at myself and see a body that I can identify with. I seem to be made up of flesh and bones, of physical matter that I can touch and feel. Yet the physicists are telling us that what we experience as solid matter is only a swirl of atoms and molecules which, in turn, are only swirls of energy with differing intensities. Is my existence an illusion and my substance a mere swirl of molecular activity?"

"Do you believe the physicists or do you believe your own experience?"

"Are you saying that it's only a matter of belief?" I said incredulously.

"No, no, Karl, it's a matter of giving priority to experience, rather than to scientific theory. It has to do with trusting your own experience, rather than with trusting the molecular theories created and taught to you by others."

I wasn't sure that I entirely understood what he was getting at and fell silent. At least he seemed to be listening more seriously now. . . . My eye caught a particularly graceful pattern of activity in the swirling flames - a waving yellow and orange fan with a tinge of blue on the edge. The glowing fan danced as the blue played a game of "hide and seek" along the edges of the orange core. It was a magnificent sight!

It suddenly struck me that it wouldn't be so bad if all I was, was a beautiful swirl! Perhaps, in his wisdom Carl was right and my original question did reflect a useful insight. . . . But now he's talking about experience. That's strange. It almost sounds as if he is resorting to claims of objective knowledge.

"Carl, I thought you were a constructivist! What is this talk of giving priority to experience? You're beginning to sound like an empiricist! What ever got into you?! Do you have a fever or something?"

I reached out jokingly to feel his brow. But he pulled away and chuckled.

"Yes, yes, I know. Most of these systemic people think that I'm a constructivist. Furthermore, to distinguish me from some of the earlier constructivists like Piaget, some of them even pinpoint me as a *radical* constructivist like von Glasersfeld. But I think I'm closer to being a bringforthist."

"A *what*?!"

"A bringforthist."

"What on earth is a bringforthist?"

"Actually, I hate being labelled with any such words. Sticking labels like constructivist, empiricist, bringforthist, etc., on people makes me squirm. But it seems to be the only way we can talk about each other and our positions when we get into the abstractions of epistemology and ontology. So I'll accept the description for now, as long as you agree that it's only for the purposes of this conversation."

"O.K. That's fair enough."

"Well, in accepting the description of being a bringforthist, I am trying to set myself apart from the looseness and extravagance of radical constructivism. It troubles me when constructivists get carried away in their solipsistic reveries and talk as if just about anything can be constructed in our distinctions."

"Yes, I know what you mean. I also feel uneasy when some therapists rely too heavily on constructivism. Sometimes they generate alternative descriptions of clinical situations as if they were at liberty to construct anything they wanted. Then they have the gall to claim that their alternative is better, healthier, deeper, more accurate, or more systemic than the client's own description! Such therapy often seems disrespectful and rather wild to me!" I could feel myself getting quite worked up about the issue.

He seemed to sense my frustration. "You see Karl, I am in agreement with Maturana that we cannot honestly construct just anything when we make distinctions. We can only bring forth into our awareness and our descriptions that which is consistent with our lived experience."

"But isn't that what von Glasersfeld calls 'fit'? The construct fits the experience like the key fits the lock?"

"Yes, but von Glasersfeld focuses primarily on the viability of the construct. He doesn't explain how the construct arises in the first place. He simply takes the observer as the generator of constructs as a given."

32

I had to agree. "Yes, the constructivists' constructs do seem to come from nowhere. . . . By the way, where did you get this idea of being a bringforthist?"

"Maturana is the main originator of bringforthism. He offers a heuristic explanation of the phenomenon of observing and of how the observer arises. He also explains how observations and constructs are brought forth in language and in consciousness."

In my reading of the literature about Maturana, he seemed to be presented as a constructivist - at least this was the case with those who wrote about him. "I thought Maturana *was* a constructivist."

"He claims he is not, and I agree with him. There is much more to bringforthism than simply generating constructs that can be used to 'fit' our experience."

Now I was getting really curious. "Apart from the broader scope of Maturana's theory to include biology and evolution, how does he differ from the constructivists? . . . Could you give me a specific example?"

"Well now, let me see. . . . O. K., von Glasersfeld tends to focus on the construct and its viability while Maturana attends not only to the construct and its domain of existence but also to the viability of both. That is, Maturana assumes a simultaneity in the bringing forth of 'figure and ground' whenever a distinction is made. Any particular distinction or construct cannot stand alone; it needs to have a context or domain of existence if it is to be brought into our experience with any degree of coherence and authenticity. The construct has to experientially fit its medium in a complementary manner before it can come into existence in the first place, and only then can it be applied to fit our ongoing experience. In other words, bringforthism demands a multiple fit in one's experience."

I was a bit puzzled. He seemed to be referring to experience an awful lot. "But doesn't this emphasis on experience begin to get rather close to empiricism?"

"Not in my mind. But I suppose it depends on your understanding of empiricism. As I understood it, the empiricists assume that there is an ontologically separate and real world out there. As a bringforthist I don't make that assumption. Instead, I assume that the world that I distinguish is actively brought forth by my own actions and, hence, that I am always inextricably part of it. The empiricists maintain a separation between the observer and the observed. They claim that as observers we can apprehend the world passively through our sensory perceptions. Furthermore, they assume that this 'real' world can be known with confidence and with certainty."

"Isn't that a rather old and naive version of empiricism?" I asked.

"Yes, but most people live according to that view most of the time."

"That's probably true but you must be familiar with some of the more recent philosophical developments that grew out of classical empiricism and which support modern science, like logical positivism." I felt that Carl was being a little unfair in his critique of empiricism.

"Yes, the logical positivists are more sophisticated. . . . Although they still assume a separate and real world, they acknowledge that it can never be known with certainty. In contrast to the classical empiricists, they only claim that our knowledge *approximates* the real world. But they have a serious problem, too."

"And what is that?"

"In my opinion, they do not realize that embedded in their notion of approximation is the implicit assumption that it is possible to *know* when one description is closer to reality than another description. What is overlooked when one uses this covert assumption is that one must have some kind of prior knowledge of the 'real world' before one can make the judgment, that one of two differing descriptions is, indeed, a closer approximation to reality than the other. As a bringforthist, I am content to relate one experience to other experiences when trying to explain something. I do not resort to any separate objective knowledge of the outside world. I think it is potentially dangerous to assume that we possess such knowledge about the world."

It was fascinating to hear him articulate the inconsistency in the logical positivist position so clearly by disclosing the underlying assumption. "But why is it dangerous?" I asked.

"Because it leads us back to the same objectivity and certainty of the naive empiricists. And, as you know, explicit and/or implicit claims of objective knowledge are used regularly to impose one's will upon another and to justify all kinds of violence in doing so. Hence, I prefer to avoid making truth claims derived from any sort of empiricism that is grounded in objectivity."

I thought he was getting a bit smug in what he was saying and wondered how he could be so sure about his own stance. "But how can you ground yourself in experience and claim *not* to be an empiricist or a positivist? Maybe your bringforthism is just another, more subtle form of empiricism." And before he could answer, I went on to proclaim: "Aha! I can see the headlines already! 'Carl von Auer's bringforthism: A new form of closet positivism'!" To my surprise, my tone seemed a bit sarcastic and confrontational.

There was a loud explosive 'snap' in the stove at that moment. It was followed by a burst of sparks and a dramatic flare of flame. But the fire didn't distract him and he was swift in his response: "Now you are being unfair, Karl. . . . I thought we agreed that I would only accept the label of 'bringforthist' for the purposes of this conversation."

He then turned away and looked into the stove. I could see from the reflection of the fire in his face that my confrontation had triggered some pain. I began to wonder if our dialogue was at risk. In reviewing what had happened, I realized that I had slipped into objectifying him as a person. I did this by assuming that he was making an objective reality claim about himself as a bringforthist rather than just using that description as a reference point. Thus, his claim about the dangers of objectivity became a case in point at that moment in our conversation. By adopting an 'objective' view of him and his

35

descriptions, even momentarily, I had endangered our discussion. . . .
An apology was in order.

"I'm sorry. You're right, I was being unfair. It just seemed that you
were so clear about your 'bringforthist' stance that I began to think
that you held it with certainty. Maybe I was confusing clarity with
certainty."

He seemed to accept my apology and actually seemed a bit
pleased that I could see the difference between clarity and certainty.
I was relieved, but still not satisfied. I still couldn't understand that
Carl could give experience so much authority without implicitly
resorting to some sort of 'real' world out there. I also wasn't quite sure
how he saw himself differing from the new radical constructivists.

But never mind. What was of greater concern to me was how I
could understand myself. Why did I experience myself as existing as
a concrete entity even though the idea of dynamic process appealed
to me so much? And if I was constituted by pure process, where did
that process exist? Was it reasonable for me to expect Carl to answer
my questions? He seemed to be drawing upon Maturana's framework
a great deal. In fact, it almost seemed that Carl von Auer and
Humberto Maturana were soul brothers! I too was attracted to
Maturana's ideas about knowledge and existence. . . . I began to feel
a new set of associations bubbling into my awareness. . . . "Carl, do
you remember a few years ago when I was so excited after I first heard
Maturana's explanation of 'mind' as a social phenomenon?"

"Yes! I too was pleased to hear his explanation of how we become
observers of the world and of ourselves through language, and how
languaging arose in the recursive coordination of actions among us.
For a long time I have felt that as human beings we bring the whole
of reality, including ourselves, into existence through our conversations. But I could never have explained it as systematically and
clearly as Maturana did." Fortunately, he seemed pleased with the
change of topic.

"Well, around that time I began to think of my 'self' as an
internalized constellation of conversations about 'Karl' which
originated in external conversations among others. In other words, I

began to think of my 'self' as first existing in the social domain of languaging rather than in my body. By thinking of myself in this way it became possible for me to begin to feel free of the physical boundaries of my body. Sometimes it was like I was outside of my skin!"

Carl laughed as he put his hand on my shoulder: "So you became a disembodied spirit for a while?" . . . The firmness and warmth of his hand felt good to me. It was nice to have some physical contact.

"Yes, the significant 'I', the person that I really experienced myself to be, just didn't exist in a physical sense at all. In fact, in those days I used to say 'I don't exist!' and I felt liberated in doing so. I loved the feeling it gave me."

"So what exactly was your 'I' that was making the claim that you didn't exist?" He smiled and gave my shoulder an encouraging squeeze.

"Well, the 'I' and 'Karl' are linguistic distinctions in a network of conversations that make up my identity as a person. I presume they originated in conversations that initially took place around me as I grew up in my family. With time, the distinctions about 'me' eventually became internalized within me. 'I' became a node in the network and I started making the distinctions about myself."

He smiled approvingly as I continued: "And since the context of these conversations per se were not material, the meaningful 'I' really didn't exist in the physical world at all! I existed in the domain of the conversations that constituted me. Furthermore, thinking about myself in this manner turned out to be a way that I could sort of transcend my physical being."

"It sounds like an exciting realization!" There was a tone of genuine excitement in his voice.

"It was!"

"Did this realization make a difference to your experience of yourself as a person?"

"Oh yes! Having discovered this pathway to what seemed like a kind of personal 'transcendence' I now set myself on it from time to time when I feel constrained or trapped. Doing so seems to open an enormous amount of space for me as a person and adds life to my life!"

"Fantastic!", he exclaimed.

I was delighted that he seemed so thoroughly enthusiastic about the idea. "And besides, during the times that I can enter into such an understanding of myself, I feel very closely connected with other people in the world. For example, I feel inextricably tied to all those persons who have contributed to the specific conversations that have brought forth the distinctions of 'me' as 'Karl' and 'Karl' as 'me' and thus brought me into existence. It really feels great to be so profoundly connected to others in one's most basic and fundamental identity!"

Carl was beaming from ear to ear. "I'd call that having a systemic 'high'!"

"It certainly is! . . . Sometimes I even get so 'high' that I feel like I am floating above my own body!" Indeed, it seemed like the conversation about it was beginning to entice me back into interpersonal space and get me a bit high.

Carl became thoughtful. He looked into the fire for a while and murmured, "Humm . . . an out-of-body experience."

"Perhaps. But such extremes only last for a short time. I can only reach such heights when my thinking is crystal clear and my emotions are free. But whenever some physical necessity arises, such as the need to walk home, to eat, to wash, or to get dressed, my physical body immediately re-emerges as the primary locus of my experience."

Carl smiled: "It almost sounds as if there are two separate Karls!"

I felt a slight pang of pain somewhere in my being. "Yes, that is exactly what is so confusing for me. There do seem to be two of me: one located in the social domain of conversations, the other in the physical domain of mass and energy. The one has a familial and cultural history, the other has a biological and phylogenetic history."

"Are you struggling with some sort of mind-body split?"

"I really don't know. I don't experience myself as being split, even when I'm feeling 'high' and almost out of my body. In my ongoing lived experience there is only *one* of me. But in my reflections there seem to be two."

"Perhaps the split lies in the dual explanations you give yourself about the physical and psychological aspects of yourself."

"Yes, that's it! Differing explanations! But how do I get them together? How does one connect a swirl of molecules and energy, with a swirl of conversations? Or do I exist in different domains simultaneously? And where does the single integrated experiential 'me' exist?" My voice had become plaintive, almost pleading. I finished my series of questions as if I was imploring him to provide me with a comprehensive answer that would tie it all together.

Carl slowly turned towards me and leaned forward. The light from the fire was quite faint by now. The earlier blaze had died down and only the red embers were still glowing. Yet I could still see well enough to notice the corner of his left eye begin to swell with a big tear. "But Karl, an explanation never replaces the phenomenon being explained anyway. An explanation of your 'self' may add to your understanding of 'self', but it can never become a substitute for your 'self'. Furthermore, your efforts to search for closer connection with your experiential 'self' through a logical explanation might only serve to distance you even further from the desired experience."

Suddenly, everything in my mind stopped. It was like I had been arrested in mid-flight! The futility of my demand for an explanatory answer became painfully apparent: my intellectual question served to preclude the experiential answer I sought! The insight moved me emotionally and I became tearful. Carl moved closer and gently put his arm around my shoulder.

He spoke comfortingly: "I once experienced a similar struggle and gained some measure of relief when I gave up striving to understand more than what was possible for me."

What came over me just then is not clear but I began to weep. Tears began streaming down my cheeks as if a water tap had been turned on. It wasn't sadness or despair. It seemed much deeper than that. Carl seemed to have tuned-in to me at quite another level and I was able to tune-in to him. It was as if our experiences began resonating. I felt totally immersed in love. I put my arms around him and we embraced one another.

It was a long and speechless moment. My original struggle simply dissolved. The experience of my being was solidly grounded in his; and being in the experience felt very good.

A few minutes later when I stood up to open the stove door and throw in another log, I felt integrated and whole - as if Carl was simply part of me and my mind and body were floating together! . . . There wasn't much more to say just then. So we both sat and watched as a new flame took hold and another undulating dance began.

Carl Auer (C. A.) and the Temptation of Objectivity

Josef Duss von Werdt

C. A. was the very incarnation of self-referentiality. Self-referential subjects are world-centers. To realize themselves as such, they have two alternatives, that of the subjective or relative - I am the center of my world or that of the objective, the dis-sociated, the absolute - I am the center of the world in general. C. A. chose the first, the ascetic alternative, and this is why he was so quickly forgotten and we have so much trouble rediscovering his traces. During his lifetime he was already considered not to be objective and thus could only become notorious rather than famous. He was laughed at, spied upon, not taken seriously, particularly in his capacitiy as a scientist, where after all he ought to have been the epitome of objectivity. But he could not de-mean himself so far as to mean only those things that would be accepted by the common mean of his fellows.

The second alternative is the more comfortable one; whoever embarks on that avenue can be sure of the back-handed, double-tongued applause of the multitude, which finds secondary narcistic satisfaction in being totally - not to say in a totalitarian manner - colonized by the objectivity of others coming from the center of the world.

Some fragments of C. A. have come down to us in which he reflects critically on Descartes. Unlike the latter he was not gulled into confusing epistemology with ontology. Thought for him was not proof of his existence but its very precondition. One of his really rather banal principles was: "Everything I think is thought by me." Flying in the face of the Cartesian axiom he wrote down the following: "Cogitata cogitans cogito cogitantem," or "Thinking that which has been thought, I think the thinker." He loved to take words literally and to explore their original meaning. Cogitare is reflexive, derived from co-agitare secum, carrying something around with one, turning inside oneself, reflecting, pondering, also meditating. Another version of that same axiom was: "Observata observans observo observantem," or "Observing the observed I observe the observer." Observare has to do with observantia, with obedience, obeisance, observance, fidelity, confidentiality, safe-keeping.

Thinking and observing are mimetic processes. They hug the wall, they do not leap over it. Mimesis judges that which is ergonomic.

Thus C. A. was of course making ethical demands of himself that bordered on the superhuman. If in all thinking and observation, I bethink and observe myself, then I am both subject and object at one and the same time. Without this kind of objectivity vis-à-vis myself, without the duality of subject and object, I can never attain selfhood, i. e. awareness of my own self. I have to put myself in a metaposition with regard to myself in order to say of myself that I am a subject.

Furthermore, there can only be objects for subjects making up together the oneness of awareness. Consciousness becomes self-consciousness, being becomes conscious being, selfhood becomes conscious selfhood. Being as such is not existent in its own right, it is the product of consciousness. A subject turning object to itself goes dual, puts distance between itself and its self. The fashionable term for this is "meta-position," a position which we normally only expect others to assume. Kant and later Husserl were talking about the same thing when they postulated a "transcendental self" which observed the "empiric self" in its dealings with itself, other selves and other things. From its position as a second remove it concerns itself with the relation between the observing observer and the observed object. Thus the transcendental ego is peering at the little egoist egging itself on to fabricate its own world. It is its own Big Brother, the authority responsible for everything that goes on between the empirical self and its objects. I am answerable for everything that I think, find, invent, do or do not do, even if I call this science and am subjecting myself to its rules. The insight that the reality of art, science, money or politics is invariably nothing other than the reality discerned, discovered or invented by the artist, scientist, economist or politician, transforms all objectivity into subjective fabrication, for which everyone of us is personally liable. Thus I cannot hide behind "science" as if such a thing actually existed in its own right, a convenient replica for reality.

For C. A. the causality between being and thinking went in the opposite direction to Descartes. What he saw to be the Cartesian error was the vision of the thinker instituting himself into being by dint of his thinking, in other words epistemology degenerating into ontology. Not "cogito, ergo sum," but "esse est; ergo sum; ergo cogito." Being does not become being through thinking. It is, however, invariably, "being for us," thought being, and thinking becomes the accomplishment of being, its co-agitation, a coming-to-self without ergo. Being is action, accomplishment, perceived and perceiving reality, which is not to say that it is what it is by dint of perception, or that it originates ex nihilo from perception.

Of course it would be convenient if we were not only the creators of our world of knowledge and actions but if this would represent the sole reality outside of ourselves. And indeed we usually act as if this were in fact the case, by positing objectivity as such. Then there would be no hunger, no hardships, no prisons, no A-bombs, no pollution. It would all depend on how we looked at things. There are, of course, those objective people for whom everything depends on the point of view and on their personal needs. Because this view is free of any kind of valuation, positive or negative, nothing is objectively evil or reprehensible to them. On the contrary. We are doing fine, objectively. We are not only at the center of the world, we are the center of the world.

Without realizing it, C. A. did in fact work out a General Theory of Relativity with reference to what human knowledge is capable of knowing. Whether Einstein knew of this is impossible to say. At all events, he never admitted as much, although it would certainly have done nothing to detract from his undeniable originality, particularly as C. A. was never bothered about such things anyway.

Although a self-referential person through and through, C. A. was no solipsist imprisoning himself in his world. He was responsible for himself alone. He identified with what he said; indeed, in terms of his objectivity, i. e. with reference to himself, he had no other choice; after all he was the one saying it.

This gave many of his contemporaries sufficient grounds to doubt his sanity. Surely this was not "normal." Only objectivity is normal, regardless of C. A. Normality is in the last resorts a question of statistical majorities and self-imprisoned constraints. Catanoic, however, i. e. according to his understanding, C. A. proceeded on the assumption that man can only possess understanding of things within the framework of his own subjective referential system (and the scientific reference system is only one of many). But as soon as he attempts to understand something without taking himself into account, he becomes paranoid. "Objects of thought dissociated from the thinker are the essence of madness," we read in another fragment.

One essential criterion affirming that he understood himself as the center of his world and not of the world is to be found in his remarks on the understanding of others, the "Thou" problem. One of his fragments reads as follows:

"You are a subject"is an ontological statement under epistemological restriction. The ontological side consists in the fact of my necessarily conceding to you an existence dissociated from me with the same claims and requirements as I have for myself. The epistemological restriction lies in the fact that 'you' become an object when I become aware of you. You become an object in me, the observer, the thinker, the artist, the therapist, the doctor. . . . I do not create you, I perceive you. You are, of course, independently of my perception, but for me you are the person I perceive. What you are for yourself I cannot know. Even if you tell me, I still cannot perceive you independently of myself. It will always be I hearing what you say. And even if I repeat what you say it is I myself doing so and it then takes on my meaning and my significance.

Here we have that decisive warning not to confuse objectivity with neutrality, not to neutralize, indeed neuterize, objects, not to treat them like so many articles and handle them as if we knew who and what they are.

Objects in C. A.'s understanding are not solid bodies, not value- and meaning-free facts but visible, symbolically, audible, with the senses perceivable *moments of encounter* with oneself as well. When I encounter you, I encounter "you in me," not myself alone and yet myself as well, not you alone, and yet you as well. Thus objects do not become a-historical, they have their temporality too. They take place, are in a state of flux, come and go in time. They are not just there, they are infinitely multiple, different for each and everyone of us. Either they are internal materializations in the subject or they are nothing. Objectivity is thus a concretely structured subjectivity. When it is taken for the truth, in a dissociated, absolute, dis-embodied sense, then this happens at the dictates of one or more subjects claiming absoluteness for themselves by the same token. Instead of something being whatever it is for me, it then becomes something of itself. This kind of objectivity is the basis of all fundamentalisms and the primal form of violence. Then science does away with religion, for example, and religion denies the validity of reality as postulated by science because it represents a danger to its own version, etc. The fact that objectivity can also be a form of intellectual indolence, or indeed arrogance, comes to the same thing. Objectivity as we know it is of course very reassuring once everyone has got accustomed to it. Politicians, for example, are very highly dependent on habit becoming the objectivity of as many individuals as possible. Only he who in no way disrupts the habits of the indolent has any chance of success. And only the successful can be in the right, i. e. objective.

Effects were made to get C. A. into politics and for a time he felt not only an external impulsion but also something akin to an internal compulsion. Inwardly he felt drawn towards political activity by the respect he had for the "subjectivity" of every individual and the commitment to ensuring that it be given due heed. Many of those who encouraged him felt that here at last was someone who would fight for politics with a human countenance. He however was subjective enough to realize that such people only had their own interests at heart, that this was an attempt to monopolize the idea of "humanity." Again and again he was brought face to face with the fact that it is all but impossible to be both a consistent relativist and at the same time to relativize the absolute necessity of being precisely that. Thus he finally decided - and this again was an outsider's decision - to remain faithful to science. For him scientia was synonymous with con-scientia, that form of cognizance that transforms science into conscience. The question of whether this kind of con-science was compatible with politics he left open. He had enough trouble with his con-scientious colleagues, most of all with those for whom scientia was largely indistinguishable from pecunia. Pecunia non olet, money does not stink, in other words it too is value-free.

Nobody really knows what became of C. A. This habit of his of reducing himself to his initials may lead us to suppose that he did not set any great store by his own person. Nor do we have any indication whether he ever toyed with the idea of embarking on a course of psychotherapy. It seems at all events highly probable that he was urgently advised to do so, for the approach was still a very novel one in his times. But all the same, objectively speaking, who else could possibly have been more in need of it than people like C. A.?! On the other hand with his personality make-up he would probably have had difficulty in finding an analyst. He was constantly forgetting himself and thus lacked that essential instrument of analysis, the ability to recall, to retrieve those deep-frozen products, those objective "facts" and things of his own little history.

If we look around in world history in search of like-minded scholars and philosophers, three major figures immediately spring to mind: Laotze in China, Heraklitus a century later and another century later Kratylos, in Greece and Asia Minor. All three have something in common. They left us a legacy of wisdom, left it in the truest sense of leaving it behind them while they moved on into unknown realms, into regions where nobody would follow. It is said of Laotze and Heraklitus that they, as it were, took themselves out of circulation; they simply disappeared. Kratylos relativized Heraklitus' own relativity ("You cannot get into the same river twice") by insisting that "you cannot even get into the same river once." Thereafter he withdrew into himself, made signs with his little finger if there was anything he urgently needed but aside from that never opened his mouth to speak again. All of these resisted the temptation of objectivity; their legacy is the annoyance they caused. The way they were constituted represented a certain kind of ethics that made spoilsports out of them. For in this sporting life it is objectivity that is the great gambler, putting everything at stakes, life, mankind, air, genetic structure, spirit, mind, the Earth. To all this objectivity does violence.

If our sources are correct those three pre-Christian philosophers did not look upon themselves as specialists in a particular subject. Laotze in fact would probably have said that a "subject" can only emerge when there's nothing left of substance to talk about. C. A. was so supremely ethical that he was not even self-righteous. It is for this reason that he remains like a thorn in the flesh of our thinking - come to think of it, a pretty successful "survival strategy" for someone outwardly so unsuccessful!

46

Auer as Smuggler[1]
Carlos E. Sluzki

I never knew whether to believe him or not. I still don't. Perhaps that is an effect intended by him . . . if there is any intent of effect at all! Perhaps that is an effect regardless of intent, a moral of the story conveyed by the great scheme of things. Well, all this convoluted prologue is my feeble attempt to delay my wish to share a startling revelation - if revelation at all - and an incredible story that Carl Auer poured over me during my recent visit to his cottage. First of all, it was April, and you know how Aprils are, neither here nor there. Secondly, he might have been a bit tipsy when he mentioned it to me (one never knew whether that sturdy mug filled with tea-mit-Schnapps which accompanies him whenever he is at home retains miraculously its fluid - theory #1: Carl is a closet teetotaller. Ridiculous! - or is consumed and re-filled again and again throughout his endless evenings - theory #2: Carl is a closet alcoholic. Nonsense!). I don't even know whether his revelations were to be kept secret, a tender confidence that I am shamelessly betraying by writing this, or perhaps general knowledge that only I came by tardily. And thirdly, perhaps I misunderstood the whole tirade: the conversation took place too late at night - too late for me, a morning dove, but not for Carl, definitely a night owl. You see, I am at my best at 6 a.m. and tend to decline progressively throughout the day, becoming a mumbling idiot at 6 p.m. and a total zombie after dark, body present and soul in suspended animation - while Carl is just the opposite: he barely manages to struggle to the kitchen in pyjama and robe, grab his double, nay, triple expresso swiftly prepared and handed to him by whatever tender guardian angel - that is how he calls them - is around him (and how does this rather conservative-looking old man manage to secure those silent, attractive, almost etherial guardian angels around him. This seems to me to be another act of magic!), drags himself to the bathtub, unable to mutter even an appreciation, only to reappear an hour later looking refreshed but still as if drawn with *mezzatinta* and *sfumatura*, and becomes progressively alive as the day goes by, to bloom at night in a blinding display of intellectual pyrotechnics, frequently witnessed only by his cat (and whatever female guardian angel may be floating around), sometimes solely by the somber presence of whatever remained of Bertha after the well-known mishap, and, alas, sometimes just by him and his old battered Olympia, much to everybody's delayed benefit.

Well, the whole thing started during one of those nights by the fireplace, just the two of us, when Carl told me, in the middle of a conversation, almost mumbling to himself while looking sleepily at his filled mug: "You know, Carlos, I never ever read a book in my life."

I managed to shake myself from catalepsy and answered, following a social mandate that recommends that when one utterly doesn't understand something, one has to transform it into something understandable, regardless of how banal: "I cannot believe that you didn't like *any* book in your whole life!"

"I liked *many* books! What I said is that I never *read* one."

"In what language?" I insisted, trivializing in order to make sense of it.

"In what language what? In what language didn't I read any book? In all kinds of languages! That is, I didn't read any book only in those seven languages that I know. Needless to say, I haven't even *tried* not to read books in languages that are unknown to me."

He is pulling my leg, I decided, he is teasing me benevolently, perhaps because he notices that I am half asleep and wants to flip me into an altered state, as he has been known to do now and then. I remember drawing at that moment a flash comparison between Carl and Gregory Bateson. Well, there's a difference if ever I've seen one, I thought. If Gregory saw you meandering, and even if not, he wouldn't pull your leg, he would simply fly higher with the effect of making you feel like a wingless insect, he would mutter something abstruse to assure that you would be lost, no pebbles to follow him through the clouds, his flying coordinates hopelessly above and beyond your reach. And don't come to me with any positively connoting metaphor about the Buddhist master and the transcendental nature of the incomprehensible: Bateson didn't mind being cruel. But not Auer. He may occasionally be a teaser - I told myself, and still believe - but his mischievousness is always tinted by the warm colors of his kind soul. I managed to shake off my sleepiness and attempted to probe in which direction he was meandering: "And what about all you have written?"

"But, Carlos," he threw his arms up in (mock?) despair, "we are not talking about my writings! It's nothing to do with my writings, really, I just follow the blessed advice that André Gide offered me once. It happened, let's see . . . it was Paris . . . yes, I remember, in 1949. I was lamenting to him the pangs of inhabiting the body of a person for whom creativity is a core value and therefore is condemned to expect daily of himself what occurs only by miracle - as you see, a variation of the 'be spontaneous' paradox. Gide stabbed me in the chest with his bony index finger, then shook it in front of me as if to prove that it was still intact, and admonished me with his high pitched *falsetto*: "*Mein freund*" - that was the extent of his German! - "everything has already been written and said before! But since nobody listens or remembers, we have to keep going back and beginning again. We don't write, we only re-write! And that is what I do, Carlos, I re-write. Only as nobody remembers what the other have written, I am called 'original'!"

A mantle of sadness enveloped us and tinted the silence that followed. God, was I awake! And ready to cry, at what I wasn't sure. And Carl seemed equally moved, a genius condemned by his own wisdom to re-writing, even when the most original pieces were pouring from the seemingly bottomless well of his creative mind. "Well, Carlos," he seemed to extract himself from the quagmire by pulling himself up by his own bootstraps, *à la* Munchhausen, "after all, true sculptors only chisel away the excess granite in order to discover the finished piece that lies hidden in the rock."

The lifting effect of that idea was instantaneous: to define Michel-angelo as a discoverer rather than as a creator, or perhaps as a chamber-boy that meticulously dusted away with his chisel whatever pieces were hiding a pre-existing, already formed *Pieta* seemed so ludicrous that my somber mood faded away as quickly as it had come. Stubbornly, I returned to my track: "Carl, I distinctly remember your quoting almost verbatim, not too long ago, in one of your Heidelberg lectures, some passages of the *Tractatus Logico-Philosophicus*. Where did you get that quote from, if you didn't read it?"

"*Wovon man nicht sprechen kann, darüber muß man schweigen*. But, why not, it was so long ago . . . Do you want to know how I quote it? Let me tell you, Carlos," he mumbled, his eyes closed, while rolling up his sleeve to show me his left forearm, which was decorated by a rather ugly flat remnant of an old wound, one of those pinkish, melted-cheese-looking, scar-over-scar-over-scar things, the size and shape of a fossil giant trilobite. "Do you know where I got this tattoo? It comes from the very last days of The War To End All Wars (he pronounced each capital letter distinctly), where I volunteered - for the wrong side, of course, meaning by that, I guess, 'for the side that lost it' - when I was fresh from *Gymnasium*, too young to know any better. Anyhow, in October 1918 I ended up with a piece of shrapnel in my arm and was taken prisoner by the Italians - and don't ask me which side the Italians were on: I still don't know, and they probably didn't know either. I was sent, wound and all, to a prison camp near Monte Cassino. And there a miracle occurred: prisoners were distributed in cells not according to rank, nor to age, nor by alphabetic order, but according to still another equally silly bureaucratic parameter - could you believe it - place of birth! And I ended up sharing a cell with a total stranger, a fellow prisoner in that camp. It was, Carlos, of all the people in the world, Ludwig Wittgenstein. I must confess that I had never heard of him - I recognised his family name, of course, as his father was a well-known industrialist in Austria. He was many years my senior, 30 years old, while I was . . . well, still a toddler. Can you believe it, Carlos, Ludwig, bursting with ideas, carrying in his jacket at all times the only copy of the manuscript of his *Tractatus*, re-working it daily, making it tighter, clearer, cleaner, but in a desparate need of a dialogue with peers, stuck in a cell with this *ignoramus*. However, God bless him! rather than cursing the gods - or worse, cursing me! - for his fate, he made from the start what could be defined as the most desperate or the most genial move in that terribly constrained situation: he carried me conceptually, he taught me meticulously from the very basics to the very frontier of his own thoughts - imagine, Carlos, Wittgenstein by Wittgenstein! - in the hope of making of me somebody he could learn from. In turn, I, being as I was almost *a tabula rasa*, and totally unaware that his was an impossible task, immersed myself into this work with devotion. And this irritable, hyper-sensitive man, prone to mood swings and at times unable to exorcise the dark clouds that followed him, was consistently warm and endlessly patient with me. I, in turn, was stubbornly receptive. We would converse incessantly, from dawn to dusk, in the cell and in the yard, alone or surrounded by fellow prisoners. The guards were probably convinced that they were dealing with a pair of lunatics and treated us accordingly: they left us in peace. He would explain his propositions again and again - '*Die Logik muß für sich selber sorgen,*' he would mutter stubbornly - and I would also argue again and again until I understood, and then continue arguing until we both understood that I understood. In fact, in those four months of endless conversations, many parts of his manuscript were re-written and re-written anew. Mind you, it is not that I was such a genius, it was simply that here and there I seemed to ask the right questions to force some revisions, and was able to provide here and there the right alternatives that allowed for new propositions to be formulated.

Ludwig ended up referring to it, bless his soul, as 'our' manuscript. My! for me it was a daily miracle. Those months have been, Carlos, by far the paramount intellectual *fest* of my life. Ridiculous as it may sound, the most cherished period of my whole existence took place in that cold, rotten, prison camp. But, as in all stories, suddenly, one morning the unexpected occurred (and it occurred on a Wednesday, which is a good day to expect the unexpected): during early roll call, one of the prison's wardens appeared, medals and all, and informed us, in broken German, with the unavoidable seasoning of Italian epithets, that he was carrying good news, 'even though you, *rompescatole*, always complaining of cold and hunger, don't deserve any': all prisoners who were 18 years old or less were going to be pardoned and released immediately. The screams of joy were deafening - there were many adolescents, caught by the war machinery as 'dead meat of last resource' that managed to land in the camp. Ludwig and I looked at each other's eyes for a seemingly endless lapse, flabbergasted, tears cascading freely down our cheeks. We then hugged each other in what felt like a lovers' soul-tearing departing embrace - I am sure that many fellow prisoners in fact thought that there *had to* be some suspicious hanky-panky between us. Then, with an urgency I had never heard in his voice, Wittgenstein whispered anxiously in my ear: 'This is our chance, Carl. You have to take this risk for me.' I didn't know what he was talking about. He went on: 'You *have* to smuggle our manuscript out of Monte Cassino. You have to take it to the British Embassy and urge them to send it to my teacher, to Bertrand Russell, - I believe he is now at the University of Peking. I *need* his feedback. I have gone as far as I can go and even further thanks to you, my beloved friend. But I need Russell, I need to hear from him. I may not get out of this camp ever!' His sobbing made his words almost unintelligible. 'Tell me that you will do it, tell me, Carl, please!' His distress was overwhelming: it was no longer us, dear friends, master-disciple, saying good-bye, it was a desperate father pleading for me to save his baby from certain death, an artist urging me to rescue his masterpiece from a sinking ship.

All along I had been soothing him - and I meant it, mind you - 'Of course, Ludwig, of course,' but he seemed to need to finish his tirade. It took me a while to realize that, while talking, right there, in the middle of the noisy crowd on the prison's chilly yard, surrounded by cheering youngsters and somber adults, in what seemed an awkwardly extended embrace, he was pulling out surreptitiously his - our! - manuscript from his jacket - where he carried it constantly, priceless treasure as it was - and pushing it with despair into the inner pocket of my jacket. In fact, I realized later, that maneuver had to be done there and then, in that moment of confusion: we, the youngsters, were *ipso facto* bathed, shaven, given clean clothes, and ushered to the train.

Anyhow, I managed to smuggle it away. After fencing off countless secretaries and attachés, I was able to deliver it in person to the new British Consul in Vienna. The manuscript reached Bertrand in Peking as planned, he was in turn able to write to Ludwig at Monte Cassino, courtesy of the Red Cross, Ludwig then wrote to me, I wrote to Bertrand, and so on and so forth. The rest you probably know. So, summarizing, how come I have been able to quasi quote the *Tractatus* without reading it? Because I participated in some minor fashion in *writing* it, that's how, and because I discussed it inside out with its (main) author! So stop asking."

So stop asking! On my behalf this man was displaying incredible archeological artifacts from his own history - from the collective history of our culture, in fact - and then dismissing them as obvious with a flippant "So stop asking." I brushed aside his comment, my mind in turmoil and awe. I remember that at that moment the enigmatic dedication of the first edition of Wittgenstein's last book, *Philosophische Untersuchungen*, crossed my mind: "To C. A., student,

53

mentor and smuggler." The first time I saw that inscription I already suspected that "C. A." had to be Carl Auer. But why "smuggler"? I had my question answered.

The dance of the flames in the fireplace suddenly came into focus at the end of that story. I allowed myself to sink into the warmth of the fire and of the moment, mesmerized by the vibrant silence that followed, like an aftermath, that privileged incursion through a time warp. After a while, still in trance, I asked Carl: "And have you ever returned to Monte Cassino?"

"To Monte Cassino? No! In fact, I couldn't, even if I had wanted to: one can never go to any place twice, as there isn't such a thing as places that stay while time and oneself, the visitor, evolve. In fact," he interrupted me just when I was starting to cry mercy, "not long ago I heard Ludwig's nephew Heinz[2] presenting a variation of what I told him once, which I will repeat for your benefit: one can never visit a place *once* - Heinz transformed it into 'one cannot cross a river once,' but that's because he doesn't want to get wet, hein? It's late, Carlos, I'll go to bed now, if I may. Thank you for accompanying me in my story. Make yourself at home, you know where the bar and the bathroom and the guest bedroom are if you wish to stay - it's rather chilly outside. One way or another, to be continued."

Once again, there I was, dizzy from the effects of another punch into my mental plexus. "Just one quick question, just a 'yes' or 'no', Carl. Does your 'never having read a book' and your 'being unable to go to a place once,' or twice, or whatever, belong to the same gender?"

Auer looked at me, faintly smiling, his head slightly tilted. "It's late, Carlos, don't torture me," he pleaded.

Sucker for human rights as I am, I dropped the issue and bid him good night.

[1] Chapter 7 of Carlos E. Sluzki: *The Re-drawing of the Jigsaw Puzzle: Fireside Conversations with Carl Auer*. New York and Heidelberg, Neueman Verlag, 1990 (in press, bilingual edition). Reproduced here with permission of the author and the publisher.
[2] Heinz von Foerster (the editors).

Proofs

Carl Auer and the Ethics of the Pythagoreans
Heinz von Foerster

I am, of course, delighted that Carl Auer, this extraordinary, strange and extremely creative man, is at last being commemorated by this Festschrift. I am particularly grateful to the editors of this Festschrift for giving me the opportunity to present Carl Auer with my thanks for the strong influence he had on me in his early youth. Let me tell you how I met and got to know Carl Auer.

In my youth the Austrian school system was organized in such a way that all children started primary school ("Volksschule") at the age of five or six and stayed there for five years. After finishing primary school they moved up to the secondary school ("Mittel-schule") for a further eight years, after which they could attend college, either university or technical college. I started primary school at about five years of age and spent the first four years at a state school. I was one of the worst pupils. To be more precise, I was not only *one of* the worst pupils. I was maybe even *the* worst pupil. I well remember having to sit at the very last desk. In front of me, at the last desk but one, sat two of the many orphans who came from an institution in Vienna where orphans were interned. Every morning a few minutes before eight they came marching along in their striped - horizontally striped - prison clothes. Their heads were shaved so that not even a few lice could stray onto or into their heads. Dieter Medwed, one of these pupils, sat in front of me, and he really didn't know the answer to one question. Yet I still had to sit behind him, for sometimes I knew an answer, but it was generally considered to be "impudent". On these occasions the teacher, Mr. Holzinger, would come towards me smiling kindly. He would twist the hair growing behind and in front of my ear together and pull me up by this hair, so that I had to climb onto the bench and then onto the desk to make me understand my impudence.

I didn't feel very happy in this school, so my parents decided to transfer me from primary school to secondary school a little earlier than normal. This was possible, but one had to take an examination if one wished to go to secondary school after just four years in primary school. The problem was, however, how could I, such a bad pupil, survive or pass this exam, the centerpiece of which was in mathematics. As I wasn't really that bad at math, my parents thought a few hours extra tuition would enable me to cope with the curriculum required for the exam. Thus it was suggested that a young man come to us as private tutor. His name was Carl Auer. He was recommended to my family as he was said to have been a very bad pupil too. He had failed several times and had had to repeat a year or two, but he was known to be very good in mathematics and physics. So it was that Carl Auer came to our house and began to prepare me for secondary school.

I had a lot of fun with this young man who not only knew a lot, but was also very interested in what interested me. I remember well that I was particularly interested in a certain mathematical step: the idea of proof. Carl was particularly skillful in introducing me to the "proof." We began with my having to prove the Pythagorean theorem. Carl introduced me to this proof by demonstrating the proof Socrates showed Menon. As you may remember, Pythagoras' theorem consists in proving that in a right triangle the sum of the squares above the two legs, a, b, namely $a^2 + b^2$, is equal in area to the square which can be drawn above the hypotenuse: c^2. This results in Pythagoras' theorem: $a^2 + b^2 = c^2$.

Socrates' proof consists in drawing squares above the hypotenuse and over the two legs in an isosceles right triangle (see Fig. 1), and showing that the area of the two small squares (each consisting of two isosceles right triangles) corresponds exactly to the area of the large square over the hypothenuse (consisting of four isosceles right triangles). I was so fascinated by this illustrative proof because I understood what it means when one 'sees' something: the idea of insight. One suddenly says: Aha, now I see how these relations come about. When you have understood this proof of Pythagoras' theorem for an isosceles right-triangle it is no longer difficult to understand this method of proof or a similar one for right triangles in general.

Fig. 1

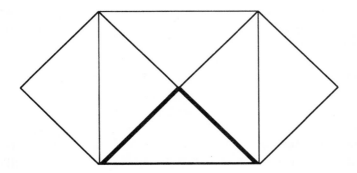

Carl Auer soon realized that this young boy had easy access to graphic and geometrical problems and that this shouldn't be exploited too far, but he should rather be given insight into algebraic relations. And so he taught me that, apart from these fascinating geometrical relations between a^2 and b^2 and c^2, there are also interesting algebraic relations. That, for example, there are whole numbers such as 3, 4 and 5 that have Pythagorean relations, namely: $3^2 + 4^2 = 5^2$. And that this relation not only exists for 3, 4 and 5, but for many other triples, such as 5, 12 and 13 or 7, 24 and 25, which all have in common that the sum of the square of the first two numbers equals the square of the third.

These mathematical somersaults were great fun. And when the time came for the examination I passed with no difficulty at all.

A few weeks later I was admitted to the secondary school. As was the custom at that time, each new pupil was introduced to the headmaster of the school. So I went in too, and the headmaster said: "You passed the math exam very nicely. We are happy to have you here. Who taught you math?" Proudly I replied: "Mr. Carl Auer." At that the headmaster immediately slapped me. He grabbed me by the ear, lead me out of the room and showed me the school's large yard. From there one could see that almost everywhere streaks of black ink had been smeared over the stone walls of the building from the windows of the third floor. And he hinted that these ink spots had been made by Carl Auer when he was a pupil of this school many years ago. He remarked: "Should you have learned characteristics other than those of a mathematician from your Carl Auer, I would advise you to get rid of them as soon as possible."

In spite of the headmaster's warning I continued my relationship with Carl Auer and went to see him evenings, or he came to us. We spoke about mathematical proofs of other problems.

One day I asked him: "Tell me, Carl, you introduced me to Pythagorean numbers, where you square two natural numbers and the sum of these two corresponds to the square of a third number. Are there higher powers, so that, for example, not only a^2 plus b^2 equals c^2, but maybe a^3 plus b^3 equals c^3. Are there any numbers, a, b, c, which fulfill this condition?"

He became very serious after I had asked this question. He kept absolutely quiet, then after a few minutes he said: "You have touched on a big problem that a great mathematician postulated 200 years ago. His name was Fermat. Fermat gave this problem a lot of thought and finally came to the conclusion that there are no such numbers. He reported the fact that he had come to this conclusion in the margin of a book in which this problem was posed. It must have been a text book on the theory of numbers in which Fermat wrote in the margin: "I can prove that for no exponents, n, larger than two are there three numbers $a^n + b^n = c^n$ so that this relation is valid for whole numbers. Unfortunately though the width of this margin is too narrow for me to set out the whole proof on this page."

During the 200 years since Fermat touched on this problem - it is generally referred to as "Fermat's Last Theorem" - ever more mathematicians have tried to work out this proof for themselves, but no one has ever succeeded. Such unsuccessful efforts of proof are, of course, a fascinating stimulus. And I asked myself straight away: How can Fermat's theorem be proved? And I asked Carl too:

"Now tell me, have you ever tried to prove this theorem?" For a long time he said nothing. Then he nodded and said: "Yes, I have tried." - "And, have you proved it?" - "Yes," he said, "I've proved it." - "Then why don't you publish it, for heaven's sake? Then all the mathematicians who have tried so hard to prove this theorem would be relieved at last!" - "Yes, I've thought about it a lot," Carl answered, "but I have decided not to publish it." - "But why not?" - "The proof could be written in the narrow margin of this paper." - "But that's .... Why don't you publish that too?" - "Fermat knew that too, of course," Carl replied, "and if he didn't want to write this proof in the margin of that page, then he must have known why this proof should not be written down. Who am I, Carl Auer, to write this proof down when Fermat decided not to?"

This ethical attitude of Carl Auer's impressed me deeply. Not until much later did I realize that it in fact corresponds to that of the Pythagoreans, who did not wish to impart their deeper insights to others unless they were sure they could not lead to social abuse. One not only finds this ethical position implicit in constructivism, but also in Ludwig Wittgenstein's *Tractatus Logico-Philosophicus*. Proposition 6.421 reads: "It is clear that ethics cannot be articulated" ("Es ist klar, daß sich Ethik nicht aussprechen läßt"). That is, that at the very moment when one starts to talk "ethics", one begins to moralize. Then one always says how the *other* should behave: "*Thou* shalt" or "*Thou* shalt not!" But ethics is concerned with one's own behaviour, one can apply it only to oneself, i.e., you say to yourself: "I should" or "I should not!" That cannot be said to anyone else, you can only say it to yourself. Just as one can prove Fermat's theory for oneself, just as one can have many insights for oneself. The only thing one can do as a constructivist is to give others the opportunity to construct their own world. I think I owe these insights to Carl Auer's understanding, comprehensible and mild way of talking to me when I was a small boy about mathematics and its insights.

Carl/a Auer: An Invention
Donald A. Bloch

My recollection of Auer as you will see is ambiguous. But it may help to knit up the strands of others' memories.

Students of this fascinating life have assembled such varied remembrances that one might, the historical evidence notwithstanding, believe that Carl/a Auer is a fiction, a dream figure in our collective dream. It is hard to think of anyone who would be more amused by this than Auer and at the same time who would take it more seriously. Auer might well say that if we think we have dreamed him, perhaps we should think again, maybe he has dreamed us. Or, more soberly, dreamed himself.

My life intersected with his in 1948. Just back from a year of internship I was a new, very young and very eager resident at the Chestnut Lodge Sanitarium, a psychoanalytic hospital set in the lovely rolling countryside of Maryland, just outside of Washington D.C. The Lodge had rapidly evolved in those post-war years into a flourishing intellectual nursery. I have often wondered why, since Chestnut Lodge (or The Lodge as we all called it) was an unlikely site for this flowering and Dexter Means Bullard an unlikely leader.

In any case, the Lodge had existed in its previous incarnation as a drying out spa for alcoholic Congressmen and other illustrious residents of Washington D.C. Following the close of World War II the city was in the early stages of a transformation from a sleepy post-Civil War small town into the glamorous world capital and suburban sprawl it would become in the next decades. Dexter Bullard, who had inherited the Sanitarium from his father, chose to change its character as well and make the hospital into a world capital of psychoanalytic treatment for schizophrenics and other seriously disordered folks. He infused the hospital with the bizarre notion that one could treat such patients with intensive psychotherapy or psychoanalysis. Bullard was guided in this by the quirky American genius Harry Stack Sullivan and by the brilliant European psychoanalysts and philosophers he had imported before, during and immediately after World War II.

Frieda Fromm-Reichman was the most illustrious of this group. I believe she introduced Bullard to Auer, whom she had known as a brilliant colleague before her flight from Germany, but I may be wrong about that.

Rumor had it that Auer had worked on some kind of wartime cryptoanalysis device. Perhaps he had been a collaborator of Turing on the Enigma machine. We were never to know although certainly the term Enigma was appropriate for him. The notion of breaking obscure codes appealed to us as we tried to understand the language of madness.

As young psychiatrists in training we were possessed, drawn into the phantasmagoric fields where our lives and the lives of our patients intersected. This was particularly true at the "Lodge" since the notion of the interpersonal field was a given. Psychometabolic rates were unimaginably high. Most of us suffered from the *furor interpretandis*; all of us were driven to be therapeutically successful, as therapists and as patients, since we all were being psychoanalyzed at the same time. I recall Don Jackson and Harold Searles, who had the same training analyst, in a dry debate as to who had been *best* and who had been *most* analyzed. And (unlike now?) we believed in our current myths: the vaginal orgasm reigned supreme, the clitoris was a rudimentary organ of infantile female sexuality, homosexuality was a disease, and the dual career family laudable but unworkable. We believed in reality, even though it was the reality of Sullivan's consensual validation.

Into this steamy and overwrought atmosphere (I have not mentioned our stressed marriages, personal ambitions, and economically precarious situations nor our involvement in the psychoanalytic training wars of those days) Auer materialized. A few months after I arrived, I shall never forget that, Auer materialized. First he wasn't there and then slowly he was. Much in the same fashion less than a year later he dematerialized, on his way to Berkeley it was said.

I would say that Auer made a great impression on me and on the rest of us. He was cool and we were fevered. We were smart enough but he was, how shall I put it, cerebral. His clothing was distinctive; he favored suits that were a bit large on him and that had an unusual European cut. While an aroma of dark deeds, espionage, and double agentry clung to him, he seemed to be a totally gentle person. In some funny way he seemed to always be in soft focus; it was hard to see him but hard to know why that was so. For example, his wartime history was never spoken about and now I cannot recall how that became part of our image of him.

During the early months of his short tenure at the Lodge I tried not to notice him. His coolness contrasted unfavorably with my agitated intensity and I always found myself feeling inadequate in his presence. Towards the end, by contrast, I found myself seeking him out, as if somehow I could learn a great lesson about myself through him.

His role, if such it can be called, was to be a Scholar in Residence. Bullard was a marvel at identifying interesting talents and then letting them sort themselves out. Auer fitted into this scheme well since nothing more was required of him than to be present. It soon became clear that what interested him at the hospital was definitely not therapy. He set about conducting an inquiry into the nature of sanity.

The inquiry was finely grained, carried out by what he called "little conversations." When present Auer was always quietly speaking with one other person, occasionally a staff member but much more commonly a patient. I can still see him, elbows on folded knees, thin body, somehow swimming in his habitually oversized grey suits, intently leaning towards his "conversational companion." He would use this latter phrase to politely introduce you to whomever he happened to be speaking with, usually forgetting that you knew them. He had the ability to create a quiet private island even in a hallway streaming with staff and patient psychosis.

In those days severely disturbed patients were commonly quieted down by barbiturates, chloral hydrate and cold wet sheet packs, the wonderful discoveries of latter-day psychopharmacology having not yet been made. Auer would have his "little conversations" anywhere, in seclusion rooms or under a tree on the lawn. And at any hour. They would last for a few minutes or in one instance with a patient of mine for 26 hours. My patient was also a European, a frighteningly paranoid young man, large, blond and fierce, who barely tolerated me.

The 26-hour-"little conversation" began before dawn as the nurses informed me when I arrived at the usual time. Frederick, my patient, had been "dangerously upset" and had been wrestled into a cold wet sheet pack where he promptly became mute. When I arrived on the ward several hours later he and Auer were sitting up still in the seclusion room. (Fear seemed somehow irrelevant to Auer, although he did not seem particularly incautious.) I gather the talk had continued all the while the nurses were unwinding the sheets as if they were not there.

In each of his "little conversations" he was always the student being instructed by the patient, or even me, about something and always quietly pleased when he would "get it." Thus the next day he said to me, "Prince Frederick, (Did I know that he was a prince?) uses large primes to make code breaking difficult." Large primes, code breaking? I had an idea that Auer was a mathematician and cryptographer. (Did I know that about my patient?) Auer went on "and about the blood lines of several royal houses that I have never been able to decipher." Then silence, and "funny how codes seemed to get into it all the time." Frederick left the Lodge shortly thereafter. I do not remember if he improved, or if his family ran out of funds, or both.

Now here is the story I have been meaning to get to. It took place within a few weeks of Auer's scheduled departure from the Lodge. I was a young man in an off-again, on-again marriage, working very hard, almost always sleep-deprived and a bit giddy when the rare social invitation came along. Most entertaining in Washington then went on in private homes. This evening there was a large formal party at a diplomat's residence and I was among the social supernumeraries, invited largely because my father had been a Foreign Service Officer.

Towards the end of a long evening when I was slightly drunk, more exhausted than words can describe, but still game for an adventure if one could be had, I realized that for a time I had been aware of a woman who, through the dense crowd and the haze of cigarette smoke, kept swinging in and out of focus in the middle distance across the room. I felt erotic interest; I tried to focus. And then a totally unwanted and alien thought erected itself in my mind. I became intensely uncomfortable: the insistent thought was that the woman was Carl Auer. Such a strange thought, but I did not seem to be able to stop thinking it. Nor could I stop thinking the other thought; was this what madness was like?

I swam towards her through the crowd feeling more foolish and awkward as I came closer. But the sense that I knew her persisted. She was his height and body build. Could the mass of dark hair be a wig? What nonsense! Her manner was as unlike Auer's as could be, agitated, flirtatious, with rapid small movements, turning from one to another of the group who surrounded her, telling jokes, I guess, because I remember laughter. I edged closer. Her name? Carla, I thought I heard. Then my rising panic swept me away.

Auer as a drag queen? The idea was weird and abhorrent. Not Auer? Why did the thought persist? What was happening to me? Perhaps he was still an espionage agent; the prodromal signs of that mania could already be seen in Washington. I left, of course, but for days off and on I felt adrift, as if I had slipped my moorings. My analyst was of no help: after a longer than usual silence she mumbled something about "ambivalence" and "projection" as I remember it.

Something needed to be done, if possible. As I recall Auer was leaving shortly for Berkeley. A few days before his departure when an opportune moment presented itself, we had our last little conversation. I asked Auer if he had a sister. "No," he replied. Why was that wash of sadness in his voice. And then he absolutely startled me by adding after a brief silence, "no longer."

Confusion again, this time with an overwhelming tenderness as well, for somehow he evoked that. "Goodbye Carla," I said and gasped. There was a long silence and then he said, "You know, Don, if you are going to invent your life it is necessary not only to think it." Then he paused and smiled his Gioconda smile and asked gently, "don't you think?"

I have never stopped wondering: Had Carl invented Carla or perhaps Carla Carl? Or, had I invented both. Perhaps other contributors to this memorial can help.

Voices

David Epston

Dear Michael,[1]

I received your letter today with a copy of Gunthard Weber's request for our reminiscences of Carl Auer. I guess it's not really a surprise as Auer is a hard person to forget. Like so many people say about their encounters with Milton Erickson, his thoughts 'go with you,' seemingly poised to burst to life by the appropriate circumstances. Don't worry; such was the strange spell he cast over me that I did save our correspondence from 1985 and I didn't have to dig down too deep in my filing cabinet before I dug them up.

And what do you think of this? Coincidence? Or paranormal? Today, I met for the second time a 35-year-old man, oppressed by an obligation life-style. He told me he had been a "little less under the obligation of his obligation life-style" since we last met. He hears "voices" which persuade him that he has an unpaid debt to a friend or has left the door of a friend's refrigerator ajar. At times, the "voices" add insults such as "dummy", "cheat", "rip-off artist", "irresponsible", "careless". As he put it, "they have ways to bring me around to their way of thinking." I 'collapsed time' with him and he said that if he was convinced by his "voices" more, his own sphere of influence would contract so that in the end he wouldn't be able to escape from his bed and his "voices" would totally prevail over him. But, in reflecting on this dismal prospect, he recalled a "unique outcome." And was it unique! Keep reading!

He recalled travelling in Europe last year: "When I was troubled by my voices nagging me about things, I reached the conclusion that I should start challenging the reality of the voices - their allegations against me. When I started putting up a counter-case, I could sometimes break away from their grip." I asked my usual question: "How did you discover this? How did you make this discovery?"

He told me he had been hiking near Heidelberg and was resting at a *gasthaus*, perched overlooking the Neckar river. As usual, when he had paid for his *schnapps*, his 'voices' started harrassing him about whether he had paid up or not and he persisted in asking the waiter if he had done so. He could not be reassured. He had been travelling for so long now that he had got into the habit of talking aloud without being aware of it. An elderly man in *lederhosen* leaning on a stout walking stick was sitting nearby and finally turned to him and - in a reasonable version of New Zealand English - said: "Gidday, mate! Your 'voices' are not a matter for psychiatry. They are a matter for rhetoric - the art of persuasion." My client was taken aback on a number of counts, least of all this man's appearance. The description should have given him away but it didn't.

I was dumbstruck myself as his story unfolded. After a brief discussion (or was it a consultation), he suggested my client do the following: that he should invite them (the "voices") to attend a recording session, pointing to my client's tape recorder. When my client queried their willingness to accept his invitation, the man advised him to incite them by acting like a "bad boy." He said that my client might consider that the "voices" had something of importance to tell him. He proposed my client then record them into what he called "your little machine" and then submit them to close scrutiny, especially their rhetorical aspects. My client had little knowledge of rhetoric so the old man, thanks to a classical education, assisted him at some length. He then advised him to tape his own "voice," a voice that presents "your counter-case," as he called it. These are my words but the old man said something to the effect that he imagined his "voice" would argue again his further submitting to obligation and its side-effects. He said: "Give voice to your advocate's voice and tape it likewise." He then proposed that he study his "case" for a free life, free from the impoverishment of obligation and always measuring up to others' expectations.

I don't know why I am going into such detail because the important thing was that this was so close to the conversation I had with Auer on my way from Christchurch to Auckland in 1985. Remember, you flew directly to Adelaide and we parted company in the airport. It just had to be old Auer and when I checked some details, sure enough it was. What do you think of all this? What do you think of Auer's "therapy"? You know what they say about Auer that "once met, never forgotten." Auer's life is like a Dickens novel in its dependence upon coincidence. Flabbergasting, is it not?

Yours Auer-ly,

[signature]

PS: Find enclosed my letter from Oct. 9, 1985.

Dear Michael:

A remarkable thing happened on my flight to Auckland. I was pretty weary after the workshop as I imagine you were.

As is my custom, I had planned to bury myself inside some headphones and rock-and-roll myself home. I had an aisle seat. An elderly, 'foreign' man excused himself and pressed past me. I had no interest in making contact with anyone after the workshop but there was something about him that attracted me. He looked old but acted young. His eyes were vivacious and when I couldn't suppress my curiosity, I guessed by his leather satchel full of weighty books that he was on Oxford don here on sabbatical. I started sneaking glances at him which wasn't hard to do as he seemed quite in a world of his own. A DC-10 was just another university carrel to him. He vigorously slashed his way through a manuscript with a fountain pen. I remember thinking that I hadn't seen such an antiquated pen in use before.

He seemed to satisfy himself in regard to his editing, sat back and pulled out, of all things, Bateson's *Mind and Nature*. I couldn't contain myself any longer and thought I might start up a conversation with him. I did the usual opening airplane gambit. "Have you enjoyed your stay in New Zealand?" His reply baffled me on two counts: first, he spoke with quite a reasonable New Zealand accent and second, he said: "As an anti-positivist, it has had a special significance to me. But it was nothing like arriving here in 1942 with my late friend, Karl Popper. We both had secured Junior Lectureships at Canterbury University where we weathered the storms of the war years." He then enquired if I knew who Karl Popper was. I indicated I did and that was all it took for him to commence lecturing, much like I am told Wittgenstein used to at Cambridge. More or less, I became a witness to him having out loud a conversation with himself. Aphorisms were followed by oracular riddles, several of which he attempted to solve, much to his own amusement. I didn't quite know what to make of all this, so I remained attentive. I thought to myself that this wasn't rock-and-roll but my mind felt like it was getting a dry-cleaning. Abruptly, he discontinued his discourse and said: "Tell me the story of your life, young man - or would it be better put, 'story' your life's story." Without any opportunity to try a reply, he broadened his question by further musing, chaining together a number of unanswered questions:

"How does one render events or episodes out of the flow of lived experience? How are those events construed as a story? How is storied experience warranted? Does one tell one's story or is it told? What would become of a person whose story was "untellable"? What if people's lives were considered to be 'texts' and how would it be different to be a 'reader' or an 'author'?" One question seemed to breed another. It didn't seem important to him to stop and try to find an answer. I am not at all sure I understood a word of this although it was pleasing to consider how this man's mind was working. All of a sudden he snapped out of his intellectual reverie, fixed me with intense interest and asked me what I did for a living. I was caught napping and said: "Family therapy." Assuming this would make no sense to him, coming from Europe, I qualified my remarks with ... "something like psychiatry." He laughed: "Voices," he said, "they worry when people hear voices. Their question is badly put - 'Do you hear voices?' A preferable question would be - 'Which of many voices is most attractive to you?' Psychiatry is like my long-lost friend, Karl Popper. Don't you think psychiatry would be better served by scrutinizing its rhetoric? Psychiatry has selected base rhetoric. Why not noble rhetoric?"

With a flourish, he placed *Mind and Nature* in my lap and insisted I should explore its contents. Well, for the first time I felt I could contribute. "Professor," I said, "I want you to know that I am a student of the selfsame book and that Bateson has had a particular influence on my colleague and friend, Michael White, who lives in Adelaide, Australia." He looked rather surprised and said that he had been under the impression that Karl Popper had "popper-ized" us. He said this was certainly the case in the universities he had visited. "Not in my family therapy," I replied. He said: "Yes, family therapy . . . I have met some family therapists here and there." He jokingly referred to his plan to climb Ayers rock the week after. I told him of your attempts to derive a therapy from the ideas of Bateson. He expressed keen interest. By the way, his name is Carl Auer. Be prepared: he's like no one I have ever met before. I hope you will offer him some of your generous hospitality. Your life may never be the same again.

Fond regards,

PS: Write back as soon as you can. Isn't it curious that Auer and Popper were at Canterbury University at the same time and I had never heard of him before. This cannot last forever, I assure you. One day, there will be a *festschrift* for Auer and New Zealand will be honored to realize it provided refuge for this man. He has had an influence on me that will only unfold over time. I hope you don't think I have gone crazy!

[1] Both are letters to Michael White, the answer to which has unfortunately been lost.

Auer Seen from a
Woman's Point of View

Vous Ne Risqueriez Rien - A Letter
Lynn Hoffman

Dear Gunthard:

Stimulated by Ernst von Glasersfeld, who of course knew Carl Auer well, I realized that my mother had met him when she was working for *Women's Wear* fashion magazine in Paris in 1929, and he was a young man of about 30. He was a small wiry person with piercing blue eyes as she recalled (she died in 1967, so I heard this story some years ago).

My mother, who was married at the time, met him at the "vernissage" of an exhibition of a friend of hers, I think Ossip Zadkine the sculptor. She told me that she was struck by this brilliant German expatriate who was also living in Paris and was studying at the studio of Fernand Léger where my mother had previously trained. Though he was at least five years younger than she was, they began conversing, found each other attractive, and he proposed that they go to bed together. She told him she was immensely complimented, but that she was pregnant with my younger sister and pointed to her stomach. She never forgot his reply, given in very bad French: "Mais c'est mieux comme ça! Vous ne risqueriez rien!" This reduced her to helpless laughter, and they ended up not going to bed but spending a wonderful evening at the Coupole, drinking Pernod and sharing anecdotes of the wonderful Paris they had come to love.

She never met him again, but occasionally, after she returned to the U. S., she would receive letters from him. She was touched at his devotion to "La Belle Américaine" despite his marriage to three women and his involvement with many others. Her eyes sparkled and her voice became especially gentle whenever she remembered

77

the conversations with him. Maybe that's why his name got stuck in my mind.

My best love to all the Auer-Friends in Heidelberg,

[signature]

Lynn Hoffman

A Recollection of Carl Auer

Peggy Penn

I grew up surrounded by the undulating, bare black hills of a coal mining town in Western Pennsylvania. If you looked at their profile from my attic window you would see a large sleeping hunchback around whom over night a toy town of grey houses, all exactly the same, had mushroomed - as though to claim this ill-starred man as the best their fortunes could tender. It was a jerry-built town made to last as long as the coal or the men who mined it, no longer. There were many of these towns and they all had names that spoke the aspirations of the people who inhabited them; Grey, Red Onion, Blow By, Acosta, etc. They conveyed a sense of despairing immanence; this moment in time is all which fortune or God may offer, for tomorrow the mine may fall in, severing lives and handicapping any future.

My father was the one doctor in town and had come directly from medical school. His only experience around mines was shoveling iron ore down the silos for the Pittsburgh steel mills; an activity required to defray the cost of medical school during the Depression. His early practice was punctuated by the mine's catastrophes. The men who worked the mines were constantly in danger of the mine collapsing and of contracting black lung disease. The union was still almost non-existent and consisted of a few absent wags who made noise about organizing, but never, in my experience living their for five years, did they repair one structure in the mine or pay for the crippling of one man.

I always knew when the mine collapsed. I heard the screaming of the women, "doctor! doctor!" I ran into the street and they streamed from between the rows of houses like a sudden flood. I stood perfectly still and they parted around me, screaming, "the doctor, where is the doctor?" Some women tore their dresses open in front, some tore at their hair, for time was of the essence; everyone must be quickly alarmed to save the men. I, too, looked for my father and often found him already running in the crowd, headed for the mine, his black bag clutched to his chest. Never sure which way to go, I usually fled into my house and sat under the dining room table which my mother told me we were so lucky to have, trying to control my violent trembling and somewhere on the verge of knowing I was afraid for my father's life. What if the mine collapsed again while he was in it? Who would save him? Who would save the rest of us and me? All night I could hear constant moaning in the small room attached to our house which was my father's office. The lights burnt all night as he treated the limbs, heads, and wounds of the survivors. I stayed awake until I could no longer smell the burnt coffee or hear the dark moaning and talking. Finally I slept praying to wake to the familiar occurrence of morning, nothing more. On the days when all was well I sat with my exhausted father at breakfast, watching him cut and chew every bite as though without my scrutiny he would not survive. But one morning all had not gone well. My father stood in his black suit in the hall, waiting for my mother to finish dressing. They told me Mr. Kapuchinsky had been hurt in the mine collapse and not survived. They were going to a church service for him. This was unbelievable; Mr. Kapuchinsky was a man whom I had helped in May and June to make dandelion wine. We picked all the dandelions we could find and put them in big vats along with orange and apple halves and special field flowers only he knew about. He prided himself on his recipe and when the wine was ready everyone in town came to taste it. They all received half a cup of wine and they toasted him, teasing him for his recipe. He would wink at me and say only he and I knew it and neither of us could write. On that day he made me a crown of dandelions and wildflowers which I kept until the fall when it turned to brown dust. After my parents left I went to his house and looked for him in every familiar place; his pipe smoking chair, his garden, and his small kitchen, but he was not present. Always forbidden to go to church alone because I had to cross the railroad tracks, today I did:

80

I could not believe Mr. Kapuchinsky was "dead." I sat on the white fence in front of the church looking through the open door and listening to the long swells of organ music mixed with crying. I decided to join the family in the church so I too could see him and say goodbye. My parents were shocked when I walked down the aisle behind the distraught family, stood in front of the coffin and said, "I looked for you at home because I wanted to say good-bye Mr. Kapuchinsky, and I hope I see you again." This was my only social farewell, taught to me by my mother.

Leaving the church ahead of my parents, I went straight to a meadow in front of the woods behind my house; stretched out in the autumn grasses like a fallen angel and floated to my secret future when I would plant my own meadow with dandelions for Mr. Kapuchinsky, but in a new town without a mine.

Often I walked to a favorite family house in a different row from ours, a Polish family house where the entire first floor was a busy kitchen. Since I was not four I couldn't attend Kindergarten and so, I prided myself on my "job" - helping Mrs. Jandor prepare the four o'clock dinner for her family. The mine whistle blew at 3:45 p.m. and supper was served in every home by four. My job was to plough with my hands through sacks of beans, picking out the bad ones and reserving only the good ones to soak for tomorrow's dinner. Mrs. Jandor put all the soaked beans from yesterday in a big black pot on the wood stove and made a fire. Then we went outside and picked "greens," dandelion greens, or beet greens if available, for flavor. If times were good, a slab of bacon with almost no meat on it went into the pot. Then she baked nine loaves of bread; one for each member of her family and some left over to pack in their lunches tomorrow. I felt such urgent directions from my stomach that I did my best to make myself useful enough to hang around until supper time when they would offer me a small bowl of beans and a piece of dipping bread. It all tasted like ambrosia to me but it was hard to explain to my parents why I didn't eat my own dinner at 5:30. They must have figured out where I spent my afternoons for my father made me a "special" sign to wear. Not sensing any villainy I wore it proudly. However, as time went by, my job deteriorated and Mrs. Jandor didn't need me so much, especially around supper time. I waylaid her daughter on the way home from school and asked her to read my sign. She burst out laughing and read, "Please do not feed!"

It was into this world at this time in my life that Carl Auer came. At first I thought he was a relative. He was introduced as a distant cousin of my mother's - a euphemism usually reserved for relationships that are hard to explain. He arrived in a shiny blue car, the only other car I had ever seen except my father's which was by now unpainted and rattled from the chains he kept in the trunk for winter "calls." But here was a car that came from an outside life I knew nothing about. I thought a lot about changing my life in those days. Now that I was almost four, I knew I would probably never be any smarter so I'd better make plans. I listened intently as my parents talked to Carl Auer. Their conversations were full of laughter as they planned picnics, swimming jaunts, drives; unheard of activities in our usual world. To the first picnic my mother wore a gauzy dress with ruffles at the hem and my father's face smiled at her all afternoon. I wanted unbearably to be my mother that summer day!

Carl Auer sat in my meadow and read to us all from a book; sometimes his eyes just focused on the horizon for a long time, other times he would catch my eye and smile with what I thought to be pure radiance. The words in some odd way, seemed shaped to fit each other, like a song. How was I to know that these young people who were my parents and Carl Auer were reading poetry. Every sentence he read filled my lungs like a bellows. The day expanded. I suddenly knew that words like these, that language, could plant fields and fields of dandelions and that language could reach into the mine to become another form of rescue for Mr. Kapuchinsky, for Mrs. Jandor, for my father and for us all. Carl Auer was a poet at this time in his life and my first friend after Mrs. Jandor.

Over the next 30 years our exchanges were usually in the form of a poem. At first they encouragingly came from him to me, but somewhere before adolescence I wrote some lines I found the courage to send. I know he lived in Europe before the war and then took his family to New Zealand, vowing never to live through another world war. At this point Carl Auer, the inner poet, agreed with Robert Bly when he wrote, "We make war like a man anointing himself."

In New Zealand he put poetry aside and pursued the life sciences, determined that the outer man must now preserve the world whatever inner refusals that entailed. But I will always be grateful to him for teaching me what Wallace Stevens cites as the difference between "things as they are" and, "things as they are upon the blue guitar."

Jelena and Carl: The Usual is Penetrated by the Unusual

Rosmarie Welter-Enderlin

As far as Carl's and Jelena's residence in our house is concerned, my opinions and those of my brothers and sisters diverge considerably. Even Jelena, on a visit to Europe just a short while ago, could not decide whether it was in 1945 or 1946 when they moved in with us. What is known, is that the Auers left for America in 1949. It was just after Carl's 49th birthday, which we had celebrated with friends of the Auers and our large family until late in the summer night under the apple tree behind our house, presumably about the middle of August. The two rucksacks they had carried on their arrival several years before were stowed in one of the many boxes, which we elder children then carted to the station. "Just in case," said Jelena, as she folded the empty rucksacks. "Who knows what use they might still be in this century of mass migration. Perhaps one day we'll be fleeing in the other direction, from West to East."

Searching for Tracks

It is well known, and yet still irritating: The experience of how differently people - in this case brothers and sisters - tell the same story. When visiting my brothers and sisters over the past few months to talk to them about our recollections of Jelena and Carl, it seemed to me that we must have grown up in completely different worlds. The kind of things we remembered showed that the pictures that have stuck in our minds can be pure fiction for others who shared the same world their whole childhood long. "You have always been known for your vivid imagination," one of my brothers said as I related my recollections of the Auers, "a real fibber. Remember how you used to tell us ghost stories at night, when we slept in the hay during the holidays, till we all actually saw and heard them? I wonder how you deal with reality professionally. . . ."

This divergence between the world of living and the world of meaning amongst my brothers and sisters and myself was painful, even at that time. The differing recollections of women and men as diverse possibilities of truth; gender as the fundamental organizational pattern of reality-construction? Is it possible that the women in our family, as in many others that I meet every day, had to develop a different memory for family history than the men? A memory that enables them to search for tracks in the labyrinth of myths and norms with their noses to the ground in order to find a place for themselves to which they are not unquestionably entitled as are the sons? Or did we simply need this different form of memory in order to free ourselves from the wonderfully luxurious yet at the same time overwhelmingly strong "family-we"? In the sense that our grass grew on the same childhood meadow, but in order to grow up we had to store the hay in different lofts? Does love mean perceiving similarities in unsimilar things and at the same time drawing nourishment from common roots for the appreciation of the differences, for the pleasure in the varied development of brothers and sisters, of men and women?

My mother's notes on the empty pages of our discarded exercise books - diary would be a much too ambitious word for it - which I discovered among her things after her death, helped me get by. In the post-war entries, for which she normally noted only day and month, the names Jelena and Carl appear shortly after the death of our Aunt Lisette, the woman who travelled alone to the World Exhibition in Paris in the last century and who was punished for it by her husband, who left her, and which she told us children without anger when she showed us a tiny Eiffel Tower she had bought with her last francs. I remember that we put an advertisment in the newspaper to let her flat in the upstairs of our old house with the remark "furnished", which was obviously a handicap at that time. For this reason the flat was still empty when we received a letter from Marie, who had served an apprenticeship as gardener with my father before the war. She wrote from Tyrol that she was looking for a flat in Switzerland for a couple they had hidden from the Nazis on their alpine pasture at the beginning of the war and who were hoping to find work in Zurich. Before the war both the Auers had been 'reds', she had to inform us of this straight away for the sake of honesty, but they were educated and very respectable people nevertheless. The fact that Jelena was Jewish and had already fled from Serbia must have tipped the scales, as my mother's notes revealed. "After all the guilt we Swiss took upon ourselves when we closed our borders and sent these people to their deaths," she wrote, "the least we can do is to say yes to this."

The fact that our parents decided this way and no other has had a sustained influence on my life. I don't know which path I would have taken without Jelena and Carl, but I do know that I am still drawing from what they both awakened in me. They came to us from a world which had been almost completely destroyed as far as its material characteristics are concerned, but they brought an intellect and culture with them which blew into our tradition-bound life in the frugality of a small town like a fresh wind. Not that intellect and culture were altogether lacking in our family. But in the struggle for existence at a time when market-garden flowers were only being bought for weddings and funerals, and vegetables had to be grown instead, my parents had lost all interest in culture. In this they were not alone. The demon of wartime and the post-war period dried up the already barren land for culture in Switzerland completely. During the war there had been pockets of resistance such as the playhouse. Wolfgang Langhoff played Brecht. He met the Auers later when he was buying vegetable seedlings for his country garden in the nursery. But after the war Wilhelm Tell was put on again, compulsory for all higher school classes, in celebration of the defeat of tyranny. People were proud of the national establishment of armed neutrality and fostered myths which promote a sense of community as the historical truth, without questioning whether the overthrown tyrant had possibly spared the country because he was impressed by the comfortable stability and the secret bank accounts rather than by the rifle in every Swiss citizens' wardrobe. And it was certainly not the case that the free democratic attitude they were virtually born with gave everyone an equal chance to start anew. It served rather to isolate the privileged from the less privileged and in particular as exterior isolation, and everything foreign automatically became displeasing. The Auers moved in in this epoch characterized by the spirit of monotony, diligence and order.

I still remember how happy I was when the rucksacks with the personal things which Jelena and Carl brought with them were followed a few days later by a washing basket full of books. Together with the typewriter, an Underwood, they were moved into Aunt Lisette's living room. Just like everyone in our family who could read, I craved anything in print. For me reading and being read to were small respites from the frugality of everyday life, meant immersion in different realities. For that very reason reading was limited to peripheral hours and to Sundays, and half an hour after the evening meal was set aside for reading aloud from the daily newspaper or the weekly magazine, whereby the feature section with "to be continued" was the most exciting. Everybody knew that the reading ban had the opposite effect, and that we children positively devoured books under the blankets or during monotonous jobs. I even caught father often with an open book next to him on the work-bench in the greenhouse, pushing seedlings into the earth with an absent look. - And so now two people who read and wrote professionally, as their job, were living under the same roof as us. This was a completely new idea, a perspective that evoked magnificent pictures of the future, ones full of other things than order, propriety and the grind in garden and greenhouses. . . .

Jelena and Carl met each other in Vienna in the editorial office of a socialist newspaper. After Austria's Anschluss to the Third Reich Carl, biologist and anthropologist, and Jelena, a few years younger and a student of Philosophy, had stayed on in the editorial office until the last moment. I don't know how they managed to get to our Marie in the Stubai Valley, but I distinctly remember my heart pounding every time their last-minute escape was talked about. At that time the Second World War was not on the school curriculum, and even in the higher classes it was only mentioned in passing, as entrance ticket to Wilhelm Tell, so to speak. So I had to piece together my own world history from scraps of grown-up conversation.

In the Beginning was the Word

At first Jelena's and Carl's words seemed artificial to me. We spoke dialect, even in school, and for us German was a written language, never a spoken one. When Jelena and Carl ate with us, which became more and more a matter of course, as they frequently gave us a hand with our work, "in order to do something real for once," as they said, I always felt as if we were mounting a stage and slipping into a new role, like actors. By speaking high German everything seemed to change colour and meaning, the ordinary became extraordinary, the world transformed itself. At first, however, we stumbled over our heavy tongues, skated on thin ice, ashamed of our clumsiness. Step by step we learned to control ourselves and to play with words, hesitantly at first, then with more and more pleasure. Even while remembering, I can still feel the excitement of the new worlds which dawned on me in conversation with the Auers, when they put names to things that had been nameless for me until then. At that time I spoke high German to myself, alone on my way to school, and told myself stories that I had never heard that way before.

Words as the key to a different reality: the Auers gave me this key at a time when I soaked words up like a sponge, infatuated with language. I can still hear Jelena's voice when she caught me with a book in the stairwell, where I was supposed to be cleaning the stairs: "Don't put blind faith in the words, child. They can make the dead rise again, but they can also kill. At your age I was as much in love with words as you. Now I have become suspicious. I have experienced what effect words can have. It isn't events that determine the course of the world, but the way we imagine them and the words with which we describe them." - The fact that these sentences have stuck in my mind has less to do with their content, which I only understood by way of suggestion, than with Jelena's attitude, which suited the way I lived at that time. The invention of reality through language, the little respites through stories, building castles in the air - "Build castles in the air, children, it doesn't cost anything, and who knows what will become of them," our father used to say, - all this was part of my childhood and was now respected and legitimized by our guests.

Carl

As time passed we learnt that Carl's works, typed on the Underwood on the top floor, were attracting attention in the outside world. Carl was given a teaching post at the Swiss Institute of Science and Technology and was only at home evenings. Letters came for him from America, and from the conversations at table it became apparent that he had published a paper that imparted a new view of biology, a new way of viewing mankind. I had no idea what that meant, but once overheard an excited conversation between Carl and our father, the hobby biologist. It had to do with father's hobby, evolution and genetics, that I remember distinctly. Father not only read anything he could find on this subject, he also told us children about it and aroused our curiosity about the purple rose he was hoping to cultivate. While we waited - in vain - and were certain that he would give it the names of his three daughters, we proudly showed our friends the five sorts of apple that he had grafted on to the "Fürst Bismarck" tree next to the place where we sat, one sort for each apple month. - I vaguely remember Carl reproaching my father for his "blind belief in progress," when my father vehemently supported his idea that mankind would naturally develop to a higher stage of morality, which would render a war such as the one just experienced unimaginable in thousands (or was it hundreds of thousands?) of years. "Just look at your much praised dolphins," he said to Carl. "They are so peaceful because their brain has had far more time to develop than that of man." I didn't quite understand Carl's arguments. I, 10 or 12 years old, only heard that he was extremely concerned when he spoke of the development of the human mind, which, due to a terrible mistake, equated progress with the destruction of the world it lived in and had now - in contrast to the dolphins - caused the basis for a peaceful development to sway. The expression "It is five minutes to twelve or later," which I afterwards heard throughout my childhood, sometimes aroused fear in me, but even more the strength to resist.

Jelena

As Carl's star began to shine, Jelena seemed strangely ill-humored. She went to philosophical lectures at the University in Zurich, wrote as well, although no-one seemed interested in printing her work. To earn money for them both she worked in the Central Library, preferably Saturdays and Sundays, as she got double pay on those days. It wasn't until later that I heard that she had helped Carl write the papers that made him famous and had then translated them into English too. She supported his scientific discoveries with the formal logic of philosophy, and together with him developed a language which was able to express complex matters in a simple and elegant way, for which he was soon to become famous.

Once, it must have been 1948, Jelena returned from Zurich very agitated. Mother and I met her on the way home from the station, and mother asked her what was wrong. Jelena usually spoke rather thoughtfully in her soft, Slavic way, but now her voice cracked."I went to visit Milena, she's Einstein's divorced wife, from Novi Sad like me, and a distant relation of my family. It's tragic the way she is vegetating in Albert's shadow. She's a highly talented mathematician! She subordinated her whole life to her husband's work, and now she's 73, alone and very ill. More in mind than in body, it seems to me, but she won't live much longer. . . . Do you know that Milena deserves a place in the history of science for her experiments in the physical laboratory and for her mathematical contribution to the development of Albert's theories? A place equal to that of her husband! And where did she end up? In his shadow, lonely, unknown, without importance. But worst of all, do you know what's worst of all? She still doesn't understand a thing, she still thinks it's natural that it's the way it is, and accepts the responsibility for her name not being included on their mutual works. She still only talks about Albert, although she hasn't seen him for years. He did bequeath her the money he received for the Nobel Prize, for he is a benevolent person. But what is that to her? And what is it to him that he never understood these correlations?"

Not until later, much later, did I understand Jelena's indignation. There was something else that united "us women," Jelena, my mother and I. In our house we only had "running cold and cold water", so every Saturday evening we had to go through the ritual in the bathroom extension, which also served as washroom. In turn we children were allowed to heat up the copper boiler with firewood and the contents of the waste paper baskets. I loved this job. As soon as the fire had caught, I would sit on the four-wheeled cart that spent the winter in the bathroom, soon cosily enveloped in steam, and go through the waste paper baskets in search of interesting scraps, looking for tracks through words, feeling for paths into the unknown; curious about the connections grown-ups never thought to explain to the child, suspecting secret stories and tying loose ends into a fabric. The "fibber" is probably not far from the truth. . . . From the time the Auers moved into our house the search for clues really became exciting. I understood little of what was on the manuscript pages or notes that were thrown away. What interested me most of all were Jelena's handwritten notes. I must have left several of them lying around, smoothed out. For Jelena's protection apparently, my mother put them in her note books, where I found them again decades later. It cannot be coincidence that she kept scraps on which I now read:

"Noted while translating Carl's book: German is a good language for the simple reason that it contains two words for the term 'reality': 'Wirklichkeit' and 'Realität.' I wonder whether both existed before Kant? Must trace it back."

- "Really nice that in German 'Mensch' is not identical with 'man.' Nice? Who over the centuries has answered the question: 'Lord, what is man?' Masters and men who were able to brood in their studies, while the other half of mankind prepared their daily bread in the kitchens. Mankind = man. Talking of daily bread: I am going to stop feeding Carl so diligently every day, with bread and with admiration, and feed myself better instead. In Rilke I read something in the *Cornet* which I feel to be a woman's poem rather than a soldier's:

Rest. Just for once to be a guest. Not always compelled to satisfy one's own needs with meagre fare. Not always grasping with hostile hands. But just for once let everything happen, and know whatever happens will be good."

Jelena, who had words for things that even my mother only vaguely suspected at that time, how thankful I am for her words and pictures! She planted suspicions in me that later became, and indeed still become, knowledge. She approved of my curiosity and doubts at a time when plain, unquestioning conformity was far more desirable, particularly in a girl. The casualness with which she dug in the soil with her hands when planting vegetables, the pleasure with which she rolled out pasta dough on the kitchen table or plucked a freshly slaughtered chicken on her knees taught me that clear thinking, provocative questioning and sensuousness are possibilities of one and the same person, provided he or she refuses to be limited to the typically male or typically female characteristics. Not that this was the easier path, either for her or for me, but whoever sets out on this path finds no way back.

A picture emerges which has fixed itself in my mind forever. One day in Autumn my younger sister came running home from school through thick fog, into the house where I was preparing the evening meal with Jelena. In tears she threw herself at Jelena. "I was so frightened," she sobbed. "All of a sudden I didn't know whether this house and all of you existed, or whether I'm just dreaming it all and will suddenly wake up and be all on my own. . . ." The abyss that opened up at such a moment was already known to me from my own terrifying experience. For we don't live in the world, but in the pictures we make of it in our heads, and children know this, even if they hardly ever talk about it and so cannot be consoled in anyone's arms, as my sister was in Jelena's that time.- Later I learnt to connect the incredibility of this image with the realization that our dreams and ideas can also imply freedom. But the feeling of the abyss that is connected with freedom remained. Possibly the only consolation for the fact that "the thing-in-itself" doesn't exist, can only really be found in the loving embrace of another person.

Epilogue

The thread between the Auers and us never snapped completely, even though we sometimes lost touch with one another for years. I met Carl once more, exactly thirty years after our farewell at our home town train station. It wasn't easy to find him in Arcosanti, in the Arizona desert, where he was planning the 'new city' with Paolo Soleri and a young Mexican architect. We finally managed to contact him through Jelena, who was living in Europe again. In Phoenix, Milton Erickson pointed out the way and showed us dozens of cast iron bells on the trees in his garden which had been cast in a workshop in Arcosanti. One of these hangs on the tree behind our house now, and when its ringing keeps me awake on stormy nights pictures well up in me, memories of the meeting with these two old men on the edge of the desert.

Carl had become famous. I read his name again and again in the works in my own vocational field, applied social sciences and systemic therapy. It's strange that a natural scientist should become a kind of saint in our territory, Carl thought so too. He had of course thought about the Condition Humaine, not only about the evolution of cells, he said, but he could provide no formulas for a better life or for how people could solve their problems.

But in spite of this he enjoyed visits from his disciples, even if this has the aura of a typical male organization about it. "Sometimes I feel quite ashamed," he said, "when a well-read young man comes to me who has accepted my ideas, sometimes quite loosely formulated, as the pure doctrine. And when he even starts making one of my essays into a theory on the essence of human beings and their possibility to change, which you therapists pack into your first aid kits as hand tools for all kinds of repair work, I can't help feeling a bit queasy. However, the people who come to you are presumably intelligent enough not to allow themselves to be patched like a water pipe. As you can see, I miss Jelena with her precise language and her superior housewife's common sense in many ways. I may be able to think systemically, but I have little aptitude to formulate systematically or to bother about the use of my insights in everyday life. This is one of the reasons I have come to the desert and am at last learning to use my hands."

Carl, over seventy meanwhile, still told stories as enchantingly as before and still permitted my questions to tempt him to tell stories. I was most interested in how he dealt with women. "They don't come often," he said with a wink. "Of course I enjoy being surrounded by willing hands, fortunately that is something that has never been lacking in my life, I am obviously the ideal father of ideal daughters. But in your field I seem to have a better reputation with the men than with the women." He didn't attempt an explanation until after his fourth Tequila: "Men like to shine in reflected glory. Maybe most women, apart from Jelena, can't believe in their own glory. They remain the great women behind the great men. Could that be?"

Jelena - "Jeländer-Jelieber," as my father used to call her somewhat adoringly, the popular name for honeysuckle (Lonicera) and symbol of loyalty, wrote a long letter from the Californian hills every summer, where she spent the holidays with Carl and the two children, Carl Anton and Nina. "You will hardly understand it," she wrote after many years, "but Carl and I have separated. We might stay that way, each in his own way, more faithful to each other than if we were living together. What has been, what we have given each other and meant to each other in the 20 years we were together cannot be lost."

Jelena has emerged from Carl's shadow, late but not too late. When almost fifty she wrote a textbook on European Philosophy in the 19th and 20th Century, from a female viewpoint, as she assures us. It has become compulsory reading for female and male students, not only in American Women's Colleges, and enabled her to look forward to an old age free of cares. Now and then she teaches as a guest at American universities, and has produced a television film with her daughter Nina on the advantages of non-coeducative women's training, where apparently far more female students take the examination for their doctorate than at the so-called integrated colleges.

Not long ago we met Jelena in Venice, in February, in front of the Teatro Fenice. Her friend Claudio had just conducted Mahler's *Kindertotenlieder* - in the dying city in which in winter, when its inhabitants are almost on their own, a vitality and happiness flares up, similar to what I've experienced at the bedside of the dying, when gradually the tremendous medical bustle becomes senseless and then there is space and time for memories. Dazed, we stood in the dusk with wet faces, and held one another in our arms, just like that time long ago, in face of the abyss. . . . Jelena, magnificently dressed in blue, her eyes still sparkling, had emerged from Carl's shadow and yet spoke kindly of him. Later, at dinner in the almost empty "Fioretta", the four of us told each other about our lives, about the children. "You're bound to laugh, but Carl Junior now writes his name Karl and is the owner of a wholesale bakery in San Francisco, where they make European pastries. . . . The only way to distinguish himself from his famous father. Instead of books, he reads the Dow Jones Index, and is happy doing it."

And now for the story, the quite wonderful story I've saved till last for you because I know how mad you are about stories: On Carl's 90th birthday his son gave him a present which couldn't have been more phantastic if he'd dreamt it. He founded an academic publishing house in Heidelberg that bears his name, the Carl Auer Publishing House. You should have seen us when we invented it on a convivial Californian night. Of course the address could only be Heidelberg, stronghold of Humanism and Idealism, vision of higher education for everyone on the other side of the Atlantic, the perfect fiction. With many bottles of Zinfandel, Karl, Nina, their friends and I created the publishing team, the chosen sons of Carl the Great, a beautiful male organization with purely noble German names. All of them highly talented, and also good looking men in their prime, each one of them uniquely creative. Of course we designed robot photos for each one and fed them to the laptop computer Karl Jr. always carries with him. Sometime, when they have broken away from Carl, which will hopefully not happen for a long time, we will publish their collected biographies, with robot photos, you can do that nowadays. By the way, after a lot of thought we gave them a female colleague, a really good woman, warm and clever, to represent the female aspect. So far as I have heard even in Europe there's nothing doing without it.

Of course, Karl Jr. keeps a firm watch on things; considering all the money he has invested, this is very important. Since he cannot supervise everything from California he's found a competent scientific journalist as manager, one with European and American roots, extremely suited to repeating great ideas on either side of the Atlantic, and madly mixed up in the nepotism of the natural and social science clique. Carl would have preferred fictitious sons to a manager, you know how romantic he is, but Junior's American pragmatism convinced him in the end."

And then all that remained was for us to drink a toast with a drop from the area around Alba: Long live the Carl Auer Publishing House!

[1] Jerome Bruner, *Actual Minds, Possible Words*. Harvard University Press, Boston, Mass., 1986.
[2] Desanka Trbuhovic-Gjuric, *Im Schatten Albert Einsteins*. Verlag Haupt, Bern und Stuttgart,1983.
[3] Rosmarie Welter-Enderlin, "Wer hat Angst vor Virginia Woolf, und vor wem hat sie Angst? Gedankensplitter zu Frauen, Männern und zum Schreiben," *Zeitschrift für systemische Therapie*, 7. Jg (2) April 1989.

On the Shoulders
of Auer

Shit Happens

Steve de Shazer

It is high time that the rest of the world recognizes the importance of Carl Auer as Milwaukee did long ago. After his first visit here, the city fathers named a street after him: Auer Avenue. It was planned as a grand avenue, not just another street, but - in keeping with Carl Auer's way of thinking - it became just a mean city street without any distinction whatsoever.

Carl Auer can best be described as an itinerant philosopher. It has never been clear whether he felt forced to travel in order to spread his ideas or his spreading his ideas resulted in his being forced to travel. Regardless, his compulsive traveling meant that he found little or no time to write except on napkins he picked up in pubs and restaurants. Therefore, although often quoted, the central ideas of his philosophy are infrequently given proper citation. In fact, credit is usually given to someone else. (Which is, of course, in keeping with Auerian philosophy.)

I first met Carl in a pub near the Marquette University campus in Milwaukee. The owner and barkeep (known as Professor Le Claire), who was born in Colorado and had worked as a cowboy (with my father) in his youth, was educated in Philosophy at the Sorbonne. Here, discussions of "things philosophical" would frequently continue - with schnapps in hand - long after the pub closed.

1. Auer's central idea can be simply stated using just two words: *shit happens*. This aphorism is now showing up in the U. S. as a bumpersticker! However 999,999,999 out of 1,000,000,000 have no idea that this is Carl Auer's claim to fame. This lack of credit is exactly

what Carl meant by *shit happens*. This idea, i. e., *shit happens*, struck me as very profound in and of itself. Little do people understand that it only takes two (2) words to rid us of the tyranny of causation.

As we discussed this most profound thought over beer and sausage and its effect on both linear and circular causality, Auer's idea became clear. Once *shit happens* human beings can only react and sometimes the reaction turns out right (*Glück = good luck*, which in the Milwaukee dialect is "good shit") and sometimes it turns out wrong (*Pech = bad luck* [in Milwaukee, it's "bad shit"]) and sometimes it turns out even worse (*Unglück = worse luck* [in Milwaukee, it's "worse shit"]). Recursively, one can only react to these reactions. But, importantly, Auer believed that a reaction does not "cause" the following reaction (or re-reaction or meta-reaction). Each reaction to some shit's happening is just one more example of Shit's Happening which must be reacted to.

2. Therefore, regardless of which way one reacts, *that's life* (another uncited Auerian principle). Life is an endless string of linear pairs:

Shit happens -> Reaction

The worse the reaction, the worse the next round of shit happens and, therefore, things go from bad to wurst, rather worse.

3. One night, during an argument about the distinction between "philosophical truth" and "scientific truth," Carl Auer startled me and everyone else in the pub by claiming, and I quote: *"An easily understood, workable falsehood is more useful than a complex, but incomprehensible truth."* Only years later, when doing therapy with a family (the eldest son was said to be schizophrenic), did I begin to understand.

4. Carl Auer's ideas influenced the humorist James Thurber rather profoundly as indicated by the "Thurber aphorism": There is not a hell of a lot of difference between a) bending over backwards and b) falling flat on your face.

5. Carl Auer once remarked to me that 20 minutes waiting for a bus was shorter than 20 minutes waiting to have a tooth pulled and that both were different from 20 minutes in bed with a woman. He said that it was not just that time was relative but that many things could happen simultaneously or sequentially or randomly. After much thought he concluded that time was very strange indeed and finally figured out the truth: *Time is only nature´s way of preventing everything from happening at once.*

6. One night, in this same pub, the discussion between us and Professor Le Claire led to the relationships between "truth/falsity" and "simplicity/complexity" and "profundity/triviality." The French philosopher pushed for an "either/or" distinction in all three sets, while I pushed for a "both/and" distinction, but Carl insisted that we were both wrong and were being stupidly dogmatic. The relationship in all three cases is "both either/or and both/and" because the distinction was false. He said that pairs of this sort were always a shorthand way of saying something profound yet hidden which can be stated in this way (and again I quote): *"It is a simple task to make things complex but a complex task to make things simple."*

(It was never clear to me when and where Carl Auer was born except for one fact: He was born in a brewery just at the time the first barrel of Maibock [of some year] was being opened.)

Conversation about Carl Auer

Luigi Boscolo and his team (Paolo Bertrando, Gabriela Boi, Paola Fiocco, Meri Palvarini, Jacqueline Pereira)

LUIGI: As you well know, our meetings take place in the office. This evening, I invited you to my home to discuss a matter of great interest: the work and life of Carl Auer whom we certainly all know, directly or indirectly.

On the occasion of his 90th birthday this year, I was asked to write something about him and his contribution to the field of systemic theory, cybernetics, constructivism. According to our model based on systemic epistemology, teamwork is the best way to reach a systemic view: six points of view are better than one.

I would like to open the discussion by asking each one of you to talk about Carl Auer, hoping that (as it happens in our therapy sessions) different punctuations by the team members will lead to "patterns which connect", as old Greg (Bateson) would say. Through this process I hope we shall arrive at a comprehensive systemic view of Carl Auer's life and work, which will finally do justice to this great man.

PAOLO: As far as I know, Carl Auer influenced, even though in an indirect way, all the most important achievements in systemic therapy. What puzzles me is the question how he managed to find such great minds who would develop his ideas. It seems he had a remarkable instinct for good whisky and talented people. . . .

LUIGI: This brings to my mind a passage from von Domarus' autobiography. He tells how his principle of identity through the predicates rather than through the subjects in a syllogism, characteristic of schizophrenic thinking, had been suggested to him at a bar in Vienna. A certain Carl told him about his eccentric Aunt Mary who, in hot situations, would claim to be the Blessed Mother because she was a virgin. That very night, von Domarus conceived his famous principle which was picked up by others as being central in the pathogenesis of schizophrenia.

There is a link between Carl Auer and von Domarus' principle as well as between Carl Auer and Bateson's double-bind theory.

MERI: Then we still don't understand why Carl Auer never wanted these discoveries to be linked to him. He even begged Bateson not to mention his name, and never told his last name to von Domarus. It's quite mysterious. . . .

PAOLO: They also say that he wrote a fundamental treatise, but never wanted to get it published. Who knows why?

PAOLA: As far as I know, he has thrown it away.

JACKIE: Personally, I recall a very strange episode. While sitting on my father's lap, in Haiti - my country of origin - he used to tell me about this mysterious white man who was in Haiti in 1949. His name was Charles d'Auer. Charlie (as they called him in town), was very loved by the vodoo priests because he had revealed to them the secret of zombification.

GABRIELA: In fact, he was a chemist. . . .

JACKIE: Yes, but until this very day the voodoo priests hold this secret which was not only chemical, but coupled with techniques for influencing people.

PAOLO: Strange! In 1951 Carl Auer was in Phoenix, Arizona, where they say he taught hypnosis to a young medical doctor by the name of Milton Erickson. And hypnosis is a technique for influencing people. Maybe Erickson does not even remember since this happened in front of three bottles of Jack Daniel's, which had fogged their mind a bit.

LUIGI: If we pass from the simple hypothesis to more general ones, I see a link between these observations. It seems as if Carl Auer prefered to operate behind the scene. He was interested in manipulating, obtaining an effect on people: he was always thinking of communication, of the indirect influence. At this point, the question of his influence upon von Bertalanffy comes to my mind. . . .

PAOLA: I am sure that Carl Auer taught chemistry in Vienna at the same time as von Bertalanffy was teaching biology.

GABRIELA: What is still unclear is Carl Auer's real thinking. We know that he has stimulated the development of the ideas he had *in nuce*. But none of these ideas were his real thinking. They are only fragments. And I believe that he never wrote for one reason: his thinking was too advanced to be fully expressed and understood. Thus, it was necessary for his thoughts to emerge from the praxis gathered by people ready enough to pick them up.

PAOLA: Among these people, there is Humberto Maturana, the Chilean biologist who got the idea of his well-known study, "What the frog's eye tells the frog's brain," when he invited Carl Auer to Santiago. As they were having coffee in his living room, Maturana noticed something odd: Auer put the sugar in a fish bowl resting on a table behind him (180° from the coffee cup). Observing Carl Auer's crossed eyes, the movement of his hand and the cup, Maturana had the brilliant intuition to turn the frog's eye 180°, so that the frog would strike its tongue 180° backwards from the worm put in front of it.

LUIGI: This led to Maturana's development of the theory that there is no difference between perception and illusion, that is, the theory of objectivity in parenthesis. A psychoanalytic interpretation could relate his theory to an unconscious defense from Carl Auer's anxiety-inducing influence. In this way, he unconsciously put Carl Auer in parenthesis.

PAOLO: What a powerful master! . . .

LUIGI: This brings to my mind how his strabism gave us the idea of circular questioning. The Milan quartet, Selvini, Boscolo, Cecchin, and Prata, met him at a conference. As we were all chatting in the hall, we noticed that every time Carl Auer asked one of us a question, the other would answer.

JACKIE: It's amazing how Carl Auer used his body to get to people. This incident happened in Vienna: while sipping a schnapps at the bar and conversing on cybernetics with a certain Carl who had a cast on his left leg, Heinz von Foerster asked him about the reason for his cast. Carl explained that he had made a jump from the second to the first floor (a jump of levels). It was then that von Foerster got the idea of the cybernetics of "the first and second floor," which became of "the first and second order."

GABRIELA: But this does not help us understand Carl Auer as a person. I think that, in order to comprehend his thinking, we should first understand the man.

LUIGI: We should get into his life's story and idiosyncrasies.

MERI: There must be a reason why Carl Auer assumed the role of stimulator and observer of a whole community of thinkers.

LUIGI: There are some wild speculations about his family of origin. For instance, they say that he was Einstein's first cousin, and that he was very jealous of Einstein's success. He knew that it was impossible for him to become as famous as his cousin. That's why he avoided expressing his ideas directly and chose to have them circulate through others.

JACKIE: There is a rumor attributing the cause of all this to the very strong, almost morbid tie between Carl Auer's mother and Einstein's mother who feared that her son could have been overshadowed by Carl's brilliancy.

LUIGI: Some say that Carl Auer was the illegitimate son of a famous Italian opera singer. His secrecy could be related to his will to protect his family secret.

MERI: There are people who swear that his mother, the famous opera singer, had been analysed by Freud. It was this "case" that gave Freud the idea of utilizing a couch!

PAOLO: But Carl Auer's inability to reveal himself because he wanted to protect some members of his family must have contributed to his existential doubts. At one point, he must have asked himself who he was and whether or not he was Einstein's cousin.

PAOLA: Really, Carl Auer was much more advanced than Einstein. Deep down, Einstein continued to think that reality existed, while Carl Auer had freed himself from this prejudice long before. He understood that "reality" was a radical construction.

PAOLO: He understood it so well that, at times, he doubted his own existence! What counts for Carl Auer is that there be "ideas" in the systems, a thesis taken up by Bateson. It seems as if Carl Auer said to himself, "Even if I never existed, my ideas would still be important."

PAOLA: He was obsessed with the idea of not existing. Also, due to his crossed eyes, he was always getting answers from people to whom he had not asked a question. He probably asked himself: "Is it really I who is asking questions or is it someone else?"

PAOLO: . . . He even thought that he was asking questions of no one; therefore, no one exists.

GABRIELA: And it was just to demonstrate his own existence that he persisted in this hard work of stimulating other people's minds. And, perhaps, his ultimate goal was to produce this book to which we are contributing, and which will demonstrate in the end that he exists.

LUIGI: Let's hope! . . . Let's hope that all these contributions will convince him that he exists. In this way, we will finally give back to Carl Auer everything he has given to us.

Milan, May 1989

Things Are Not What They Are: A Letter
Humberto Maturana

Dear Gunthard,

Mr. Carl Auer was never in Chile in my living room. The event of which Paolo and Luigi speak may have occurred in relation to Dr. Roger Sperry who is the person who in 1942 did the experiment of rotating the eye of a newt and of a frog's tadpole. I repeated the experiment as a student sometime in the mid-fifties, but I did not understand what it revealed until many years later, in 1965, when I developed my theory of relativistic color coding and became concerned with the question of cognition.

Mr. Carl Auer was a friend of my mother's before I was born, but I never met him even if I knew him as a child, which I do not know. My mother used to say that Carl Auer would say if contradicted, "Things are not as they are, and, in fact, even when they are they are not." After that my mother would add of her own: "Whatever things are even if they are not, is your responsibility."

Mr. Carl Auer must have been 26 or 27 when he was in Chile in 1926 or 1927, and he did in Chile many things that he did not do, and at the same time he did not do many things that he did. Whichever is the case, according to my mother, whatever he did or did not do, he did not do it or did it doing it or not doing it as his responsibility. And, of course, this is what you are showing by recollecting all these memories about him and his doings and not doings.

Finally, I must add that although I never met Carl Auer, I never met a person who was like him so totally responsible of whatever he did or did not do. It is for this that I admire Mr. Carl Auer and that I have been willing to reveal to you so many intimate things as I have done in this letter.

Yours sincerely,

Humberto R. Maturana

Greetings!!

Greetings!!

The Galveston Experience (We Think)

Harold A. Goolishian and Harlene Anderson

The importance of Carl Auer to our development here at the Galveston Family Institute is difficult to describe and document. We must relate a long and complex history. We were young and naive clinicians at the time we first heard of his genius. The little information we had concerning his skill as a therapist and his capacities to relate the concepts of therapy to the highest order of scientific thinking, was so superlative that at first we did not believe in his existence and thought him to be a myth like Santa Claus.

We did not hear of him all at once. Quite the contrary, it was the knowing wink, the forced indifference, and the quick change of subject from our supervisors that forced us novice therapists to realize that our mentors knew of a higher order clinician than we were privileged to know. It was similar to the feeling we often had as children when the grown-ups would make remarks that somehow seemed exciting and yet forbidden; the telling of what we later learned to be off color stories too hot for small ears. That was what it was like when his name came up or when our supervisors would tell us that they knew what to do because he had said so. What we didn't realize was that his was such a powerful and overriding wisdom that we were being protected from a force we couldn't handle.

It was not until we met a clinical anthropologist, a young protegé of Carl Auer, that we actually could permit ourselves to believe in his existence and brilliance. We were talking one day (sometime in 1956) with our consultant from Palo Alto, Gregory Bateson. We had already begun our preliminary project in family therapy and had hopes that this thinker could help us find ways of describing what to us was inexplicable: a transference neurosis was not necessary to therapeutic change. Bateson told us he once knew of a clinical theoretician and philosopher who could help us puzzle through the apparent impossibility of our finding. He told us that this "person" he knew might be our only hope and only if he was still around.

We quickly asked who this miracle man might be. Bateson told us that he had already said more than he should and quickly obfuscated the subject by deliberating about differences that could make a difference even if you did not want them to. We were excited by his wisdom about differences. A little miffed, we wondered why he talked about a different subject when he knew who could answer our pressing question. Bateson with his infinite and patient obstructionism would only smile and mutter something about *obiter dictum*. Obviously we were very excited. Somewhere there was a great person, someone who had the answer to our terrifying finding and who would permit us the opportunity to enjoy a little in the way of therapeutic usufruction.

We are somewhat embarrassed to admit our next move. Our only excuse is our youth. This was over thirty years ago and perhaps we may also be excused for our infelicitous infringement by our excitement over the use of the new therapeutic technologies, our one-way mirrors and our hidden microphones. We had already become kind of benevolent "peeping toms" for our patients so we peeped on Gregory while he was sleeping. Without his knowing it, we bedded him in our therapy room made to look like an ordinary bedroom. We watched all night behind the one-way mirror.

We do not know if you have ever had the opportunity to see a great man sleep, it is an exciting event. Each snore, each breath, and each rolling over is filled with magnificent anticipation. Did he say

111

something, what will he say next? Bateson was an executant sleeper. We were not disappointed: he talked. At first it was difficult to know what he was saying, an experience that was not uncommon when listening to Bateson even while he was awake. Unfortunately our wire recorder got all tangled. We did not have audio-tape in those days so you must rely only on our constructed recollections. Bateson was talking to somebody called Carl Auer. As we put it together it seems that he was making promises. He promised not to make the same mistakes that Galileo made. He would publish in a way so as not to offend and yet to spread the truth of a fiction of Aristotelian essences and of linear reductionism.

We were frightened and not sure what we had witnessed. At first we thought Bateson was simply hallucinating. Then we thought we were. Then Carl Auer appeared. At least it seemed that he appeared or kind of appeared. There was a major transcendental influence in the bed (therapy) room that came right through the mirror. We could begin to hear clearly even though nothing was said. Carl Auer was insisting that Bateson not make the fundamental mistake that Galileo had made. He insisted that Bateson not reduce his wisdom to a mere twenty-four pages as Galileo had done in Florence. The reference here seemed to be to Galileo's paper, *The Starry Messenger*. This was the paper published in 1610 describing Galileo's observations of the satellites of Jupiter. Bateson understood. He repeated that he would always speak the truth with regard to the distinctions he made but always in such a way that it could not be reduced to a trivial twenty-four pages.

As we talked about this years later, we slowly understood that Carl Auer, the mentor of all scientific revolutions, Carl Auer, the spirit of Kuhn, was rightly concerned that too often the great insights of science are misunderstood because of the simplicity of the underlying notions. Bateson was not to do this. We knew that Bateson had fulfilled his promise to his transcendental mentor when we noted the posthumous publication of *Angels Fear*.

But that is getting ahead of our story. We had done the unforgivable. By peeping without explicit informed consent we had violated the

112

confidential spiritual relationship between a great thinker and his source. We were despondent and moribund. Bateson sensed something was wrong when he consulted with us the next day. We confessed, expecting the worst. To our surprise, our transgression was received with kindness and warmth. It was as if Bateson had wanted to share his lonely relationship with others but was afraid to reveal the story. Now we knew.

He sat us on his knee. He had large and bony knees, and he told us this metalogue:

"Do you know what a ghost is?" Gregory asked looking away as if to hide his opprobrious response to our predicted silly reply.

"Of course," we innocently replied. We had read *Webster's* from stem to stern. "A ghost is a spirit or demon."

"No," was Gregory's immediate and amused response.

We were confused and perplexed. We had spent weeks studying the dictionary because we knew he would ask us something important and we hate to fail. "What is a ghost?" we asked in childish petulance.

"A ghost," he patiently replied, "is the opposite of epistemology."

The opposite of epistemology was not what we expected and we said so. What we did not confess was that we did not know what the word meant and could not have pronounced it if he had not said it. If it was in *Webster's*, we had not seen it.

"Epistemology," he spoke as if he were raptured, "is knowledge of knowledge. It is the sum and grand reflexive total of all the little differences that make the big difference."

"But the opposite of all these differences would be no difference," we spoke in our naive certainty.

"No," he half said as he retreated behind his big brows.

We waited with restrained patience, having finally learned to never interrupt a thinker. This was a principle which, as we only discovered several decades later, had therapeutic application when we noted that it was not good to interrupt our clients.

After some time - it was as if he had been talking to someone else - he said, "No, a ghost is truly akin to Geist."

"But what is Geist?" we asked in dismayed unison.
"Geist, ghost - it is life or rather the seat of life and therefore the seat of intelligence."
We were astounded at the enormity of the answer. Could this be it? If it was it, what was it? We sunk into a morass of complex obscurity. We had been shown the lock of life but had forgotten to ask for the key.

He let us soak in our abject stupidity until some hours later he said, "To know is to close off knowing. To not know is to know the need for a difference."

"Oh," we said, feigning brilliance.
By this time Bateson was in a self-induced Bali-like trance state. "I did not know this," he continued, "until the great mentor of all post-Copernicusian scientists, the little known Geist and Ghost of all that is ecologically error-proof, the wise old man who has taught me to struggle with failure, appeared to me in my youth. I speak of Carl Auer. He knew what I was doing when I did not. Had I known I would not have still needed to know it. It was Carl Auer who has kept alive the inspiration of the last two hundred years, the unity of mind and body. It was Carl Auer, who gave Lamarck the evolutionary theory. It was Carl Auer who gave to Blake the capacity to see through his eyes and not with them. It was Carl Auer who drove Butler to the brink of family therapy with a schizophrenogenic family. It is Carl Auer who knows what it is that we do not know and it is he who inspires me." He added, just as he was awakening from his trance state, ". . . and now he will inspire you."

"When, how?!" we shouted with impatience.
"I do not know," Gregory replied with tiredness in his voice, "Sometime, somewhere, somehow he will appear. You may not know

him when you see him. You may think you see him when you do not. You may hear him when you do not see him. You may hear him when you see him and you may see him before you hear him. It is a little like 'who is on first '(if you have heard that story)."

"Oh," we said in grave sincerity, "but how will we know the message if the medium is so unknowable?"
"I can only say that the message system will be cybernetic and transform simple linear thinking."

These were words that we could not translate and Bateson would say no more.

Since that fateful day in the mid-fifties we have often talked with and been inspired by Carl Auer (we think). Like all our good teachers we have never seen him. He has never come to Galveston but he appears to us. Rumors are that he has appeared in person to others than Gregory Bateson. Someone once told us that the expression "bat-e-son" (used by some family therapists in their pre-celtic gang rituals of hypothesizing orgy) is really using a part of a little known liturgical chant that is thought to make this inspirational genius appear. Some say he is merely a construction. Some positivists say he is real. Popper says that some day we will disconfirm him. Hoffman thinks he may be the thing in the bushes. Some rumors claim that he was once actually seen by a professor in Heidelberg and that he appeared anorectic.

There is an amusing claim that he is only a solution while others claim him to be the problem solution. Dick Fisch is reported to have used his name in a masterful strategy while he was interdicting an hallucination. Dell denies that he is the true power. Minuchin claims he is not structural. Haley thinks he is organizational and perhaps the confusion between levels of our relationship system. Object relation theorists think he may be the bad mother. Wynne hopes that he may turn out to be the original pseudomutuality. Selvini et al. are quite convinced that he is the invariant prescription. Weakland knows that Carl has never received a degree and that if he did it would be in Chemical Engineering in order to better study anthropology. Someone whose name we cannot reveal once told us with absolute conviction that Whitaker talks with Carl Auer whenever he goes to sleep in a therapy session. We were assured that whenever Whitaker goes to sleep it is to consult and open conversation with Carl Auer. Bloch has wondered if he may not be Nathan Ackerman returning to set us straight. Bowen once said that Carl is the infinite source of non-individuation. Bowen's contention is that we must seek Carl Auer out and we must differentiate from him in order to truly know. Maturana, on the other hand, is convinced that Carl Auer is a distinction in the domain of Geist that has been brought forth by our pre-Columbian structure. Von Foerster has never observed him observing him but knows he is more than a trivial machine. Varela is said to have obtained his concepts on star logic by Carl Auer's continuing reference to Galileo's paper on stars. Keeney has attempted to put him to music in the form of an Italian opera. The Norwegians are convinced that he is a reflective troll. Personal construct theorists are convinced he posed as Kelly, while the psychodynamic theorists know he was really Freud. An Australian once said that he thought Carl Auer was the paradigm lost. We do not know. For us, he is more than linear, he is more than circular, he is more than systemic, he is more than cybernetic, and he may be more than hermeneutic. We have talked with him often, we think.

We had a friend write a song once about "Galveston Oh Galveston" hoping that it would trap Carl Auer into transcendental materialistic ectoplasm. It did not work. I guess he heard it and ignored us for at least a decade. He came back, we think. He particularly likes foggy days. You can almost make him out in the mist but then you wipe your eyes and he is gone. We think you can hear his voice. When he talks, you hear through your ears and not with your ears. He sounds ontologically epistemological, a sound we can not imitate. Whenever we become desperate he helps (we think). In that with him "we do not know," we continue to make a few small differences. Perhaps someday he will favor us with a telekinetic smile and a huge difference will occur to us. The danger remains, however, that when and if he does smile, and when and if we see the big difference, it may turn out to be in the final judgment only the tautologically limited reduction to pre-Galilean social axiom and definition.

The truth is that the truth does not take more than twenty-four pages. As Carl Auer has taught us, however, nobody will believe it if it does not take more. What may be worse is that he has never indicated which twenty-four pages is the real truth.

So we are left to our conversations in the fog. These conversations with Carl Auer stimulate and reinforce our Geist and Ghost. They are never about what we know and we never know if we have it. We never know if we have heard him since we never know what it is that we do not yet know. Carl Auer is the guide that drives us on our restless search for the new paradigm. He is the living ghost that saves us from the apodictic certainty of the ordinary work of our systemic science. We have learned from our unpredictable but powerful contacts in the Galveston fog with this great meta-systematist that the universe is one big test. We have also learned that the answers are always multiple choice.

Thank you Carl Auer from your foggy friends at the Galveston Family Institute.

Gone to the Dogs

A Doggy Discourse with Carl Auer (or the Man I Think Was Him)

Helm Stierlin

I first heard of Carl Auer about 40 years ago. At the time I was studying Philosophy and Medicine in Heidelberg. There was as yet hardly any sign of a Federal Republic. There were occupied zones with the respective victors. Adenauer, Globke and Heuss were making the headlines. The economic miracle and the Cold War existed side by side. Jaspers was teaching philosophical truth to an attentive community in the University assembly hall, while in Freiburg Heidegger was still banned from speaking. Freud could be read again, but was hard to get hold of. Konrad Lorenz held lectures on the loyalty of grey geese to their partners.

The zoologist Erich von Holst, a friend and colleague of Konrad Lorenz, also lectured in Heidelberg. Along with Jaspers, Victor von Weizsäcker and Radbruch he too was one of the stars of the University. Today he is regarded as the founder of biological cybernetics as a result of his discovery of the reafference principle. It was from him that I first heard of Carl Auer. Carl Auer was a pioneering researcher, thinker, biologist, psychologist and philosopher in one. After escaping from the Nazis under great difficulties, he had emigrated first to New Zealand and was now a psychological adviser in the service of the American military government. He had agreed to give a lecture on "The appearance and reality of instincts" for a small circle of listeners. Since I represented the cultural department of the Students' Union, I was allowed to take part. But the lecture was not held. Auer unexpectedly cancelled it. Von Holst consoled me with an awkward rhyme: "One day even you will realize: The further away our Auer, the more we feel his power." My response was then: "You can only say that of God." Von Holst: "Exactly."

My second chance to see Carl Auer came a few years later. I was then studying in Freiburg. I remember: sunny vineyards, mighty, still healthy Black Forest pines, sun bathing in the Altrhein surrounded by swarms of mosquitos and croaking frogs, professors still doing their rounds as 'gods in white', me on internship in the Faculty of Internal Medicine, washing out countless urine bottles and taking blood pressures. Heidegger nearby, still banned from speaking, preparing his 'turn' (Kehre) in the peace and quiet of the Black Forest. I was studying Freud's theory of instincts, wanted to compare it with Konrad Lorenz's. What wouldn't I have given for a copy of Auer's essay, "The appearance and reality of instincts." I went to Otto Köhler, the well-known ethologist then occupying the chair for zoology at the University of Freiburg, and friend of Konrad Lorenz, for advice. Maybe he had a copy of Auer's lecture. He merely said: "Young man, a respectable scientist does not get mixed up with a swine like Freud."

At last I was permitted to participate in a symposium of ethologists, as an unofficial guest. Lorenz, von Holst, Tinbergen, Kortlandt and all the other pioneers of the first hour were present. The comparison with Freud's Wednesday conferences comes involuntarily to mind. Both involved a small group of researching outsiders, who subsequently created quite a stir scientifically throughout the world. Carl Auer was expected by this group too. He was the tip. I imagined him to be like this: A man in his mid-fifties with a kind face framed by an already greying beard, an intense and at the same time dreamy expression, who still spoke with a slight Austrian or Swabian accent in spite of many years spent in the USA, a powerful partner in dialogues, hitting the nail on the head in a flash.

Yet again the great man conveyed his apologies. He was in the country, but had suddenly become ill. (A particularly nasty form of gastric 'flu was raging in South Baden at the time. It was said to have been brought in by colored French soldiers in the occupying forces.)

I was disappointed, despondent even. Was I to miss the famous clandestine thinker and researcher yet again? I was still at an age when one is inclined to admire heroes, and in which such admiration grows with the degree of distance from the object of admiration (just as about one and a half decades later the transfiguration of Mao as a people's hero seemed to increase in proportion to his distance), yet cannot quite dispense with occasional contact with the hero altogether.

At that time my hero could only be a hero of the mind - one of the format of a Carl Auer.

My semester in Freiburg was drawing to a close. Although it was rumoured that Carl Auer was staying in the Black Forest on a health cure, I had given up all hope of seeing him. But then - just before my return to Heidelberg - I did meet him, or at least I think I met him. It happened like this:

I had settled myself down at the edge of the forest. In front of me was a vineyard. The afternoon sun was wandering to the west, towards Alsace. Dragonflies were buzzing, and I was surrounded by the smell of fresh pinewood and ripe blackberries. I had opened Hegel's *Phenomenology of the Spirit* and was brooding on the philosopher's dubiously stimulating exposition on the relationship between "master and servant." My mind was wandering. Heidegger's wisdom got entangled in Hegel's dialectic jungle: "The being being nullifies the nullifying nothingness"... And then it happened. A hard push and, simultaneously, a strong smell of dog woke me from my philosophical daydreams. As I came to my senses I recognized the disturber of the peace: a huge Alsatian, which apparently had its eye not on me, but on a fieldmouse it had seen disappearing into a hole by my side. I just saw how the dog threw the mouse, by now a mere ball of grey hair and flesh, into the air one last time before swallowing it in one go.

And then he stood in front of me in person: the man I now presume, looking back, to have been Carl Auer. He corresponded almost exactly - which surely is seldom enough the case - to my inner picture of him. He actually did have a beard, even though it was red and not yet turning grey. His expression was both dreamy and intense. And although he spoke perfect German, there was just a hint of dialect which I assigned to the Bavarian-Austrian border countries.

He apologized for his Senta. She was still young, impetuous, a hothead, but a lovely creature, and for him a constant source of important discoveries besides. I was curious and asked him about these discoveries. He then sat down on the moss next to me, and that is how my only conversation - up till today - with the man I am ever more convinced was Carl Auer, developed. Whilst we talked, Senta went on hunting fieldmice.

I do not consider myself a dog lover. We had a dachshund at home, we called him Abel Müller. He stank in spite of the periodic dog baths our parents made us children give him. During a boxing match with my younger brother I once slipped in Abel's dog shit, and had to swallow defeat and humiliation at one and the same time. Thinking of Abel, I wasn't exactly enthralled by Senta. But it was obviously quite the contrary as far as Carl Auer (or the man I think was him) was concerned. He was a dog fan, in fact he had, as I was soon to realize, chosen the dog as the animal that not only taught him things of importance about the dog species, but also about homo sapiens. It could be said: What grey geese were for Lorenz, dolphins and octopi for Bateson, for Carl Auer it was dogs. This fact should make it more understandable that my only discourse with the man I thought was Carl Auer was a discourse about dogs. I hope the reader will forgive me for limiting the following short contribution to this volume to what I can still remember of this discourse (unfortunately a little muddled).

To begin with Auer spoke about the dog as an incitement - essential to many people - to take exercise. Without my Senta or another dog, I still hear him saying, I would hardly walk for an hour in the fresh air on the edge of the forest. And like me countless other people profit from this incitement to exercise. However, one can distinguish between people who have an external dog and those who have an inner dog to incite them to exercise. It is quite likely that the inner dog is superior to the external one, as it means less dependence, more autonomy, more self management. But the inner dog can also cause problems. It can be so inflexible, so fixed in its views that autonomy is reversed to slavery. He then went on to speak about a particular kind of inner dog that only exists in German-speaking countries, namely the inner *Schweinehund*. It is difficult to find a more striking phenomenon to explain the psychology of the Germans. Just consider, I hear him say with increasing emotion, just consider the Germans' recent past. Consider the millions of German warmongers, the Nazis and their passive followers who fought their inner *Schweinehund* day in and day out, thereby forgetting to ask how a man like Hitler could make them go to the dogs. The conversation then touched on Hitler himself. Auer mentioned Hitler's Alsatian. Just a few hours before he committed suicide, Hitler got married, and the

124

dog formed part of his family. Eva Braun and the dog were both bound in faith to Hitler and were rewarded with death. Death as the reward for loyalty - that too is something typically German.

As he said that he glanced at the book lying next to me, namely Hegel's *Phenomenology of the Spirit*. He was, of course, familiar with Hegel's exposition on the subject "master and servant" and even introduced the dog here as an elucidating element. I stammered something about my difficulties understanding Hegel's remarks on the relationship between master and servant and the balance of power conveyed by this relationship. For the man at my side this was the cue to turn to the subject of the allocation of power between "master and dog."

Take my Senta, he said. I agree: I am her master and she is my creature. So far, so good. Senta shows her dependence on me, she is more dependent than a child, as her speciality is loyalty. When I am angry with her and just frown slightly, she is overcome with remorse, lop-eared, a picture of misery. But do I really have power over my dog? And do I have the pleasure of power? I doubt it. When Senta whines at me remorsefully, I am filled with remorse, too. Loyalty for loyalty. She has the whip hand for triggering guilt. When I am travelling - and unfortunately I have to travel quite frequently at the moment - the thought of leaving Senta behind, pining, unhappy, feeling misunderstood by strangers, robs me of my sleep. Insofar as I am a moral being, I feel monopolized, tied down, enslaved by Senta's love and loyalty.

As Auer, or the man I thought to be him, said this (probably exaggerating a little), an idea of the essence and meaning of relationships germinated in me, which I was to develop in my later writings. In a system dominated by doggish human relationships such as my interlocutor impressed on me, one could indeed barely make out who was master and who was servant, who was the culprit and who the victim. The deeds of one were the deeds of the other - a classic example of centripetal dynamics.

Spontaneously this brought to mind a contrary scene, stimulated by my recent reading of descriptions of travel in southern countries.

(On visiting several of these at a later time, I found my ideas confirmed): A scene with countless stray dogs romping about in sundried streets in droves, shaggy, emaciated curs, mongrels, prowling around searching for rests in rubbish heaps, some lethargic, others suspicious and vicious, all thrown into the fight for survival in a cold, competitive world. These were the outcasts, the neglected, expression and result of centrifugal dynamics.

My partner seemed to have guessed my thoughts. We, Senta and I, he said, are a culprit, victim and projecting company and are undergoing coevolution.

I pricked up my ears once again. This was the first time I heard this word, which has now been adopted in our daily family therapy language. Even today I am unable to say whether Auer (or the man I thought to be him) passed the concept of coevolution on to his friend Bateson or took it over from him. It is possible that they both created a theory of coevolution independently, just as Wallace and Darwin developed one of evolution independently.

Whatever the case may be, the cue "coevolution" inspired the man next to me to further reflections relating to dogs. Today, looking back almost 40 years, they could almost be called prophetic. The coevolution of man and dog, he said, can now be traced over a period of four to five thousand years. However, it gives me little pleasure to contemplate it. After man had first tamed and domesticated the proud wild dog, he soon made a plaything out of it. He kept to the word of God, "Subdue the earth," and subdued the dog first. He bred dogs. And what dogs: monsters with screwed up building plans, doomed to waddling and to arthrosis after just a few years, dogs with floppy ears and bleary eyes, dogs like balls of wool and smaller than cats, dilatory, clumsy, childish melodramas, and also vicious and suspicious, sly monstrosities of dogs. Whatever was required, a live toy, substitute for a partner, something to dispel loneliness, a laboratory animal, the embodiment of their unrealized lust and wildness, they bred it in the dog.

After a little thought he added: Models, so to speak, of what man will do with man in a few decades. Breeding himself, he will celebrate orgies of breeding, the progress of medicine, in particular molecular biology, will make it possible. Brave new world.

My partner was brooding further. We can also find contrasting programs in man in so far as the attitude towards their offspring is concerned: On the one hand overplanning, overprotection, over-binding, overresponsibility; on the other hand the carefreeness of mating rabbits, who think: "God will take care of it." But I fear that God - let us assume that he exists and is looking down on such quagmires of human protoplasm as Lagos, Cairo, Calcutta or Mexico City - does not feel induced to judge or repair. (Translator's note: "richten" in German can also be used to mean 'do something up', 'fix', or 'repair'. The author uses the word in both senses.)

In answer to my bashful question as to whether he spent a lot of time thinking about God, he referred me to Meister Ekkehart, William Blake and Samuel Butler. They had already said it all. Take Samuel Butler, for instance, he added after a while. He said, "The designer was the design itself"! That is something to be taken into consideration.

It was, however, difficult for me to understand this. I am still puzzling over it today. (Again I am reminded of Bateson as I write this down. Did Bateson take his idea of God as a cybernetic nemesis over from Auer? Questions upon questions.)

If I remember correctly, Auer then spoke of a planetary future in which there would be only three categories of living organisms or bio-matter: (1) The human bio-matter that had adapted to a human-made environment; (2) the bio-matter of the creatures subjugated and bred by man, i.e. the bio-matter of domesticated, zoo, laboratory animals and those bred for slaughter, and finally (3) the (dwindling) bio-matter of such creatures as rats, sparrows, cockroaches, lice, bacteria and viruses which have continually managed to outwit man in his subjugation and breeding game.

This was indeed a gloomy perspective. But Auer substantiated it by returning to his doggy theme. He said: In order to satisfy the many dog breeders and dog-lovers in our western world, the wild horses in the USA would have to cop it. They were being made into dog food. But soon beef will have to start being used more and more often too. That is being bred en masse in Brazil, on meadows that are quickly turning into steppe, where rain forests grew not so very long ago. That's where I admire the Chinese. They get along without dogs, they take their canaries into the streets instead. Instead of rearing dogs, they slaughter them young. Although - and he smilingly realized the contradiction he had talked himself into - I wouldn't have enjoyed my Senta, not even as a baby.

So you see, he said, kindly embarrassed, even I am a walking contradiction, but so is the rest of mankind. Man could be divided into two parts, by the way. Those who suffer in the face of contradictions, or who make others suffer to elude their own suffering. And the others, less in number, who enjoy contradictions. I hope you belong to this minority, or if not, that you will join it as soon as possible.

With these words he rose. Senta was still chasing fieldmice in the distance. The sun was about to disappear behind the Vosges Mountains. Auer's diminishing figure vanished into the forest. The very next day I left Freiburg. It was not only my attitude to dogs that was changed by this conversation.

The Potential of Relationship

Paul Watzlawick

My only meeting with Carl Auer was purely coincidental: 1977 on the shore of Killaney Bay, south of Dublin. It was about 5 o'clock in the afternoon and I had just finished a two-day seminar. The participants were satisfied with my pearls of wisdom and the meeting dissolved itself in satisfaction, so to speak. Tired from those long hours of work, but even more so from the long flight and the time difference from San Francisco, I walked down the narrow path leading from the hotel to the sea and sat on one of the benches along the promenade. Probably like anyone who visits this area for the first time, I was struck by its almost Mediterranean beauty: a deep-blue, calm sea, embraced by two promontories, palm trees, flowering magnolias, the soft light of the setting sun from behind, warmth, silence. One of those rare moments when we feel *in tune* with it all - and when for once the intellect is not trying to find out what that "it" is.

And then suddenly, behind me, an ugly, unmistakable noise. Somebody has started kicking around an empty can. Does this always have to happen? - Every time that, for a brief moment, we are blessed to participate in that harmony, there comes some Neanderthal man and spreads acoustic stench from his transistor radio or rapes the silence with his motorcycle or with beer cans! I wait, hoping for the noise to cease, and eventually turn my head to murder this moron with my looks - and in the fraction of a second my mood turns into its opposite. For who is kicking that beer can around is a medium-sized, black dog. Never in my life have I seen an animal play with such abandon and virtuosity, with such total joy. I watch him until my neck starts to hurt and I turn my head again towards the sea. The noise behind me goes on, just like before - *but now it is part of the harmony.* And then a sudden thought: you twerp - you manage to write learned books on the construction of realities, and when you catch yourself in the process, you are all surprised. . . .

The frail, elderly gentleman on the next bench must have been watching my face and its sudden change from icy anger to blissful delight. Oh no - now he thinks he has to start a conversation. His English has the same accent as mine, and therefore I answer in Austrian German. With this tactical mistake I really get him going. But what he says has somehow firmly remained in my memory.

"How is it possible that animals can have such power over us?" It is as if he were talking almost to himself; as if my presence were irrelevant. "I was seven years old when a stray tom cat invited himself into our house. A real beauty - silky black fur, unfathomably deep, yellow eyes. My first extrafamilial relationship object, as the psychologists would probably 'explain' it. Be that as it may, his arrival changed my world. Parents, relatives, school, priests, they all had been tampering with me in order to turn me into the person I 'should' be. The cat beat them all. With calm self-confidence he taught me how he wished to be treated, what he considered pleasant, what unpleasant. His purring, the way he rolled over on his back and stretched himself luxuriously, approving my caresses or correcting them, briefly touching my lips with his paw after having sat down on the book I was reading - no present and no demonstration of love on the part of the grown-ups came anywhere near what went on between the cat and me. Somehow he managed to take me into another world in which only he and I existed."

He falls silent, and I don't know what to say. Then: "Two years later he suddenly began to cough. There were no antibiotics yet in those days. One morning I found him dead on his little bed down in the basement." He is silent again; then in a shaky voice: "I remember that all I could think was: Never, never again must I permit myself to love like that. This pain is unbearable. - And yet, it was the beginning of my gradual understanding of the immense potential of and the inexhaustible 'realities' created by relationships. - And now, I look at

130

today's youngsters and I shiver at the realization that their 'first extrafamilial relationship object' is the home computer and their source of inspiration the television screen. . . ."

The sound of an engine behind us; a short honk.

"Oh, my taxi." He gets up; a brief polite nod: "Carl Auer - good evening." And he hurries away.

What - *the* Carl Auer?? - I should have run after him . . .

That Son-of-a-Bitch

Edgar H. Auerswald

Dear Fritz,

You can have no idea of how astonished I was to receive your letter and to discover that Carl Auer is still alive. Your revelation prompts me to share a part of my life which I have not shared with anyone except for my former analyst and one very close friend. I spent many years of my life looking for that son-of-a-bitch. There was a time when I wanted to expose him publicly - to let the world know that his concern with families and his work in that realm was a fraud carried out by a man who had shown by his behavior that he did not give a rat's ass for the well-being of families. For the past several years I have assumed he was dead.

In your letter you jokingly wrote that he might, after all, be some distant uncle of mine. Let me tell you that this is no joking matter. He is not a distant relative. He is a very close relative. In fact, he is my mother.

His name, before he underwent a sex change operation was Karla Auer. In 1924, at the very young age of 24, Karla married my father, Edgar Wald, who was ten years her senior. The two of them had immigrated to the U.S. from Germany immediately after their marriage and settled in Wisconsin. Seven months after their marriage and three months after their arrival in Wisconsin, I was born. Karla had insisted that her maiden name be included in their married name, and my father who was exceptionally progressive for his day agreed. They had become the Auer-Wald family, and this is the name that appears on my birth certificate. (Subsequently, my father, wishing to dissociate himself from his marriage for reasons I will explain, but

132

stuck with a variety of documents containing that name, inserted an "s" in place of the hyphen. I have used this name, Auerswald, ever since.)

As it turned out, Karla Auer, my mother, was an unfaithful wife. Her infidelities were particularly humiliating to my father because almost all of them were carried out, not with men, but with other women. After seven years of stormy marriage, Karla gave birth to my brother and promptly left for parts unknown. No one in my family has seen her since.

I was, I must say, luckier than most children born to such a mother. Before and after Karla deserted us, I spent most of my days in the home of my father's sister, Bertha, a young and childless widow who dwelt in a house only a stone's throw away from our own. Bertha was warm and loving, and I never lacked mothering. In fact, she was so good at mothering that, when Karla left, my anger was not profound.

The same, however, cannot be said for my father and my brother. My father was devastated by her treatment of him. His reaction to his discovery of her many infidelities was to gradually withdraw from the world of shared reality and to construct his own. In his private reality, he was a psychiatrist. When Karla left, he went public with that reality. Even though he had never received the degrees and training required to practice the profession, he ultimately rented an office, printed cards (on which he substituted the "s" for the hyphen in Auer-Wald), and set himself up as a psychiatrist. For ten years he lived in that reality with his patients. He even became mildly famous as the architect of a standardized system of psychiatric diagnosis which he called DSM 1 $\frac{1}{2}$. When, ten years later, he was discovered and taken to court for practicing without a license, his lawyer convinced him to agree to an insanity defense.

Ironically, his own diagnostic system was used by the psychiatrists who examined him, and he was ultimately declared not guilty, but insane. The judge committed him to a mental hospital where he remained until his death. Trapped as he was in his own reductionist diagnostic reality, he spent his years in the hospital developing finer and more detailed diagnostic categories. His goal was to develop a system which would allow for pathological diagnosis of all humans. He succeeded. By the time death claimed him, he had developed a decision tree leading to 480 generic diagnoses, 2021 subdiagnoses, and 40089 subsubdiagnoses.

My brother fared no better. When he was deserted by Karla the day after his birth, our father had already entered his psychiatric reality, and hoping, I guess, to create a self-fulfilling prophecy, he named my brother Normal. For eighteen years as he grew up, my brother tried valiantly to live up to that name. I shall never forget his anguish when, on his eighteenth birthday, he confessed to me that he had no sense of identity because he had never been able to figure out what Normal meant. My suggestion that he could at least consider himself a point at the apex of a bell curve seemed to be of no use to him. In fact, when I made the suggestion, he hit me. On his twenty-first birthday he committed suicide, leaving a note in which he wrote that he had finally discovered the definition of Normal and thus had discovered his identity. The word, he wrote, was synonymous with boring and his identity was that of a totally boring human being. Death, he had decided, was a better fate than normality. To this day I regret that it never occurred to me to suggest to him that he change his name.

I have always been convinced that neither my father nor my brother would have met with such disaster in their lives had it not been for the actions of Karla Auer. However, the woman who mothered me, my aunt Bertha, taught me to seek meaning in my own life and activities without excessive attention to adversity or resort to blame. It is, therefore, probable that I would have swallowed my anger at my mother and proceeded with my life with no further concern for her whereabouts, had not the following chain of events intervened.

During the years that my father was practicing psychiatry, I ran across a set of the collected works of Sigmund Freud on the shelves of his office. The inscriptions on the cover page of each book stated that they were owned, not by my father, but by my mother, Karla, and each copy had been signed by Sigmund Freud himself. I asked my father about this, but he was unwilling to talk with me about my mother, who he thought all of us should try to forget. I read these books from cover to cover, and was much impressed by them. By the time I finished reading the last of them, I had decided that I would myself pursue a career as a psychoanalyst.

Years later, in 1956, as I lay on my training analyst's couch one day, expressing my anger at my mother, I told my analyst (who I shall call Dr. P.) about the volumes of Freud's work that I had found in my father's office and that they had, in fact, belonged to my mother. Something about this revelation seemed to offend him. He not only broke his silence, but, as it turned out, he lost his cool. Actually, he mumbled to himself, but his mumbling was quite loud, loud enough for me to hear. "Too bad she never read them!" is what I heard. At first, I took this to mean that he thought she would have been a better mother if she had read them, but this outburst was so uncharacteristic of him that I could not let it pass. I told him that I had heard what he had said under his breath and had wondered what he had meant. I got no immediate answer. He remained silent until a few minutes later he announced that my time was up.

Although I thought some about this incident between sessions, it seemed of minor import. I was to learn otherwise. When I next entered Dr. P.'s office, to my surprise he directed me not to lie on the couch, but rather to sit in a chair facing him. He then told me that he had decided, after some agonizing thought, that he could not continue as my analyst. He asked me to seek out another training analyst. The reason for this decision, he said, was that he could not maintain his objectivity to the degree necessary for him to conduct my analysis. He lost his objectivity, he confessed, whenever I spoke of my mother.

Karla, he told me, was not unknown to him. She had been a significant person in his life. Then he told me the following story:

In 1937, during his own psychoanalytic training, while he was looking for a case to use as one of his control cases, Karla Auer, who had just left her husband and children, had appeared in his office, seeking analysis. The life story she presented had intrigued him greatly. She had, it seems, grown up in Vienna in Freud's neighborhood. Freud, she told him, had a niece who lived part of the year in his household. This niece, said Karla, had been her best friend during most of her childhood and adolescence, and as a result Karla had spent some time in the Freud household.

Dr. P. had brought this story to his supervisor, who, also intrigued, had urged him to accept her as one of his control cases. This he had done, and he had listened with growing fascination as Karla told him about her experience with the Freud family during her childhood. Freud's niece, Annabella, was the leader of a group of neighborhood youngsters who met and played in the basement of the Freud home. One of the activities of this group was listening to the psychoanalytic sessions that Freud conducted in his office above them. They were able to hear what transpired through a hot air vent that entered his consultation room beneath the couch. Two kinds of sessions, she told him, particularly fascinated the young eavesdroppers.

Annabella, it seems, was especially interested in those sessions - of which there were many - in which Freud's female patients spoke about their responses to the sexual seductiveness of their fathers. Freud, she said, seemed to be particularly interested in these stories, and therefore they must have some special significance. After each such session she would insist that the group discuss what they had heard in detail.

The other sessions which seized their attention were those Freud held with himself as he conducted his own analysis. Although they could not see him, they could hear him as he paced back and forth from the couch to the analyst's chair. There was, Karla reported, a mystery engendered by these sessions which the young group spent many hours trying to unravel. They observed that Freud frequently admonished himself to remember that his self-analysis could easily be ruined by something which he called counter-transference. The listeners spent many fruitless hours trying to figure out what he meant.

It was, Dr. P. reported, precisely this phenomen of counter-transference which had made Karla memorable in his life. He had, it seems, become caught up in a counter-transference web in his work with her, a web in which he had been joined by his supervisor. He had fallen in love with Karla - or so he thought - and when he shared this with his supervisor, he was told that his feelings were understandable, since Karla was a remarkable woman toward whom the supervisor had developed some familiar feelings sight unseen. (Only later did Dr. P. come to understand that Karla carried an introject of Freud, and that it was this introject that both he and his supervisor had fallen in love with.)

Unable to contain his passion, Dr. P. had severed his professional relationship with Karla and declared his love to her. Karla's response to this was to disappear from his life for the next six months. Dr. P. had not quite recovered his composure when she then reappeared in his office, now looking and dressed like a man, and going by the name of Carl. She announced that, after her initial shock at his declaration of love, she had been forced to face her total lack of response, not only to him, but also to all the other men who had made similar declarations to her, including my father. She had experienced a sudden and shattering insight. She had realized that she had never really been a woman, emotionally or spiritually. She had been a man who loved women, not a woman who loved men, and she was trapped in a woman's body. The very next day she had left for Mexico City, where she had undergone a sex change operation. S/he was, s/he said, planning next to return to Vienna where s/he hoped to become a psychoanalyst her/himself. Freud, s/he said, was within her/him, and s/he wanted to pattern her/his own life accordingly.

Carl had berated Dr. P. for not having assisted him to understand this matter in the analytic work they had done and questioned Dr. P.'s capacity to become a certified psychoanalyst. Not only that, but he had sent a letter to the President of the American Psychoanalytic Association in which he told his story and raised the same question about Dr. P.'s competence.

I think you can imagine what happened. Dr. P.'s career as a psychoanalyst would undoubtedly have ended, had not his supervisor, an analyst of considerable renown, come to his aid. In a letter to the certification board he took responsibility for what had happened. He confessed that he had been seduced by the stories of Carl's (Karla's) early contacts with the Freud family, that he had failed to recognize that Carl (Karla) was not a suitable candidate for analysis, and that he had totally underestimated his (her) capacity for acting out. He had, in fact, taken the rap for what had happened.

Nevertheless, Dr. P. told me, these events had prolonged his training analysis and thus his training for at least four years, and had cost him, therefore, at least $40,000. Under these circumstances, he said, he was quite sure I would understand why he lost his objectivity when I talked of my mother.

I began this letter by expressing considerable bitterness toward Carl Auer, but I now have to tell you that after these revelations were made to me by Dr. P. and after some additional analytic work, I felt no bitterness. In fact, I developed considerable admiration for this strange creature who was my mother. Unlike my poor brother, he was certainly not boring, and, unlike my father, while he was strange he did not seem to be crazy. And, one had to admit, he had an astonishing and highly unusual capacity to wreak havoc with those who ventured close to him. Nevertheless, I had no immediate desire to reestablish contact.

My bitterness towards Auer as reflected in my opening comments in this letter unfortunately returned at a later date. In 1959, just as I was finishing my psychoanalytic training, I had taken a job working with street kids in New York City and had discovered that, not only was the reality out of which psychoanalysis had grown unknown to

138

these kids, but also that the psychoanalytic formulations and techniques that I had learned were useless in my work with them. I had, as a result, begun to study and work with their families and had become enmeshed in the early days of the family therapy movement. The change in my thinking had prompted me to think once again about my remarkable mother, and I resolved to make an effort to reestablish contact with her (him). I planned a trip to Vienna.

When I arrived there, I looked in the telephone directory for Carl Auer. There were several listings of that name. I called them all, but none turned out to be the person I sought. I then tried to track down her family of origin. No one I talked to could remember Karla Auer. Remembering that Dr. P. had told me that Carl Auer had wanted to become a psychoanalyst, I looked under the listing of psychotherapists next. There was no listing for Carl Auer, but there was a listing for Dr. Carl *von* Auer. I called the number.

Dr. von Auer himself answered the phone. There was nothing familiar about his voice. I told him my name, and where I had come from and, not knowing how else to approach him, I asked if this had any meaning for him. There was a rather long pause, but his answer was no. I then asked him if he had ever known a man by the name of Carl Auer who had come to Vienna back in the 1930s with the intention of becoming a psychoanalyst. There was another long pause. Yes, said Doctor von Auer, he had known of such a person. He had, in fact, become a physician and a psychiatrist, but he had never been accepted for analytic training, and he had returned to the United States many years ago. Where he had gone in the U. S. he did not know. I invited Dr. von Auer to have dinner with me, but he told me that he was sorry that he could not accept my invitation because he was leaving that day for a vacation. So I thanked him and continued on my way.

When I returned to the U. S., although I had little time away from my work, whenever I could I searched for Carl Auer. I first checked to see if he was a member of any of the organizations to which psychiatrists belong. He was not. Then I explored the membership of organisations for physicians. Here I found two physicians of that name, neither of whom turned out to be my mother. Once, when in Mexico City on business, I sought out the records of her (his) sex change operation, but no one there knew of his current whereabouts. When I travelled to new places, I would routinely look up the name Carl Auer in the local phone directories, and when I found it, I would call and explore. None of my efforts came to fruition. Finally, after several years of this search, I discovered that a physician named Carl Auer who had come from Germany to settle in Louisville, Kentucky, and who, as far as I could tell, was about my mother's age, had been killed in an automobile accident at approximately the time that I had begun my search. I was unable to track down the family of origin of this unfortunate person, but I decided that he (she) must have been my mother, and I abandoned my search.

Before my search ended, however, I began to run across Dr. Carl von Auer's articles in the family therapy literature. At first, I rather liked his work, especially his articles on family role stability, but as I made the epistemological shift from Cartesian/Newtonian mechanistic reductionistic reality to new science/ecosystemic reality, I paid less and less attention to it. Ultimately, I decided that he was a Newtonian reductionist pig, and I no longer bothered to read his work - that is, until he published his seminal book, *An Ecosystemic Exploration of the Family of Sigmund Freud.*

I suspect that you can guess much of the rest of this story. When I saw this book sitting on the shelf in my local bookstore, I had one of those strange experiences of prescience. I knew without opening it what it contained. I searched immediately for his stories of eavesdropping on Freud's sessions, and, of course, I found them with no trouble. Carl von Auer was my mother, after all. Once again he (she) had betrayed me!

I immediately cancelled all of my appointments and left for Vienna, where I went directly to his (her) office to confront him (her? - Oh Shit! - him). I could not believe my ears when he continued to deny that he had ever known me. When he had me ejected from his office by the police, I must confess that I had murder in my heart. After it was all over, however, this encounter turned out to be much for the best. My quest for my mother was over once and for all. His behavior had destroyed all hope in me for a reunion, and I erased him totally from my life. At first I gained some satisfaction by reading of the furor created by his book, but I soon found that I no longer cared at all about any of it. As far as I know, he never again published in English, so I was not even reminded of him in my reading. As far as I was concerned, he was dead, and indeed, since time was passing and I knew that he would by now be very old, I assumed that he actually was no longer with us.

Now, this! Out of the blue a letter arrives asking me to participate in the establishment of a publishing company that will bear his name, and in the publication of a *festschrift* to him! I cannot believe it!

Okay. I am writing this several days after I wrote the pages above, and I have calmed down considerably. I am now able to think clearly about what I want to do about all this. I cannot ignore it, for obvious reasons. If so many illustrious people in our field see merit in your proposals, Carl von Auer must have done work that I have simply not been aware of, either because it was published in German and not in English, or because I have been psychologically blind to his continuing existence. If that is the case, I owe it to myself and to the field, to familiarize myself with what he has done and to participate in some way in this project. Not only that, but I am developing a growing curiosity. I want to hear what others have to say about my mother. You have revived him for me.

So, would you be kind enough to send me references for his work since the publication of his work on the Freud family, and, if possible, copies or reprints, too. I will write you again, once I have had a chance to catch up on his work.

Also, please be sure to send me whatever others write for you about this person. I must confess I cannot wait to read what comes forth!

With utmost sincerity

E.H.Auerswald (signature)

E. H. Auer(s)wald

P. S. Talk about synchronicity! Before I had a chance to mail the above, another astonishing revelation came my way. I have been writing a section of my forthcoming book on the epistemological shift in twentieth century science which includes an exploration of the metaphorical significance and usefulness of chaos theory. Today, in the reading I am doing to research this chapter, I ran across the work Carl von Auer has done since the days when he was writing in the family therapy literature - the work which undoubtedly led you to consider him so significant.

Until today, I did not know that he had become a chaos theorist, or that it was he who convinced the United Nations to establish the controversial World Coincidence Control Center. That idea has interested and bemused me ever since it began to receive publicity, and I have often thought that I would like to meet whoever originated it. Perhaps I can love my mother after all. Since, in the reality of the new epistemology, there is no such "thing" as a "personality," I can live with him in this reality and love his ideas!

Now What?

Carl Auer? We Don't Know Him and Don't Want to Know Him!
Interview with Mara Selvini Palazzoli and Matteo Selvini

WEBER: As you know, we've named our publishing house after Carl Auer. This man - it is said - has been very innovative. We know that he was born in the year 1900 - presumably in Austria or somewhere in the Austrian border area. We also know that Carl Auer was in Italy during his early years and speaks perfect Italian. And we know that you have also met Carl personally. Luigi Boscolo described how Auer made a decisive contribution to the development of circular questioning. Luigi told us about a conference in the early seventies during which the Milan team met Carl Auer. Can you remember this conference?

MARA SELVINI PALAZZOLI: Well, I can't remember anything about it. But as I am always interested in the causes of mental illness, I am now naturally interested to know why you are convinced that I could be interested in Carl Auer. That's a symptom. . . .

WEBER: That's just it. We would like to make a connection between you and this [1]symptom.

MARA SELVINI PALAZZOLI: You want to connect me with this symptom. But why, why . . . ?

SIMON: We are looking for the roots of systemic thinking and systemic therapy. And you are undoubtedly one of its founders. For that reason we just can't believe that you haven't met Carl Auer at some stage, since he is also one of its founding fathers.

MATTEO SELVINI: The problem is that we are a long way from inventing reality. In order to construct a reality we need something real to start from. The same applies for Carl Auer. We believe that reality is constructed from something that exists and can be established by everyone.

MARA SELVINI PALAZZOLI: ... from something that has an intersubjective truth: *one* truth. Just as everyone would say that this (points to her handbag) is a bag, for example.

So, the complete change we have undergone from the work described in *Paradox and Counter-paradox* to our present work is exactly that we are not interested in what the family thinks of itself, and that we are not interested in what stories it tells. Do you understand?

SIMON: But that means we have a problem now!

MARA SELVINI PALAZZOLI: What problem?

SIMON: Luigi Boscolo maintains that you know Carl Auer. You maintain that you don't know him.

MARA SELVINI PALAZZOLI: In my opinion, Luigi Boscolo somehow thinks I still think like him, but I don't anymore.

WEBER: Gianfranco Cecchin also told us about Carl Auer. He said he is convinced that it was Carl Auer who brought psychoanalysis to Italy.

MARA SELVINI PALAZZOLI: I'd like to emphasize once again that I have no interest whatsoever in Carl Auer.

SIMON *(Question to Matteo Selvini)*: How do you explain your mother's maintaining that she does not know Carl Auer?

MATTEO SELVINI: Well, we have a great aversion to inventing things. We have a sensitive mistrust of telling stories, and when we hear that some therapists think one must tell and invent stories. We have a sensitive nose, our stomachs rebel against that kind of thing. We have the same feeling towards Carl Auer, and that's why we don't know him.

MARA SELVINI PALAZZOLI: And I'd like to add that this is the attitude of the whole team. It could appear to be paranoic rigidity, but in truth it's not that at the moment. It's a result of the rejection of what we have done before. Let me explain in more detail: For 17 years I was a psychoanalyst and believed in psychoanalysis. Then, after reading Lyman Wynne's work on mental disturbance and family relationships of schizophrenics in 1965, I immediately stopped believing in psychoanalysis and concluded my psychoanalytical work. I am not Joan of Arc, but I could afford to do that, since I was fed anyway. My husband provided for me. I could afford these silly notions, couldn't I?

After having been a psychoanalyst, I now embraced the systemic model and worked with paradoxical methods. I was in a long manic phase, in a delirium of megalomania. Because instead of needing four years to recover from anorexia, four sessions were enough. Do you understand?

I wasn't mad. But it was a natural reaction to the long frustrations of the past 17 years, during which I accompanied my patients undergoing psychoanalytic treatment to hospital on account of relapses. The same applied to psychotics. These successes were a real triumph, even if there was also a feeling of revenge on these patients: "For so many years you've put one over on me, now it's my turn!"

Then this phase passed, because I saw its faults and its limits, and I transferred to an experimental model that consisted in giving an invariant prescription. Whether it was observed, accepted, not observed or not accepted. As a result the story told by the family was not listened to, but reconstructed from the family's reactions to the prescription.

The mother of an autistic son refused the treatment because she was deeply shocked by the prescription of telling her mother, "For you the therapy we are participating in is secret; I must never tell you anything about it." That was a clear sign that her mother was more important for her than her child. So today, after nine years of work with these families we know right away, in the first session, that the parents are not telling the truth. Why? Because they insist that their only goal is to heal their son. But this is not the truth. In fact, when we give the prescription, they immediately realize that to follow it would break up their game, so they refuse to continue therapy. This is a fact, not a story told by the family. Their real goal is to maintain their game.

MATTEO SELVINI: And that is similar or comparable to the problem we have with Carl Auer: Our goal is to reveal facts and to discover what the parents are more or less consciously trying to hide. That's why we say that the problem with Carl Auer is similar to that with the families. We are too interested in finding the recurrent phenomena in the diverse family types. That's why we can't invent them; we want to discover them, since otherwise we are not in a position to do therapy. You, on the other hand, assume that the therapist can invent freely. That's how it is.

MARA SELVINI PALAZZOLI: And now comes the difficult point. This does not mean that we think we don't construct. The human mind cannot not construct. Knowledge, even scientific knowledge, advances by means of construction.

The greatest discovery of genetic science, the double helix, is certainly a construction. But it is a construction which is much closer to the facts and can explain a number of phenomena.

MATTEO SELVINI: So, a story is constructed together with the family, but it is based only on the kind of thing that others can see intersubjectively. That means that practically we want to connect facts in the families, in the systems, that not only we can determine, but others too. By

148

means of our constructions we want to create co-constructions, to build up a story out of intersubjectively perceptible facts.

MARA SELVINI PALAZZOLI: Essentially the task or work we are now doing consists in drafting maps, very specific maps, for forming a hypothesis: If, for example, a family comes with a chronic schizophrenic child, and the child is openly adored by the father, who is very attached to it and gives it a lot of attention, and the mother rejects the child, then beware! In such a case it is usual to find that there has been a previous pseudo-privileged relationship between the mother and this child and that the mother seduced the child and used him as an anti-father but abandoned him when he failed. . . . Or when a sibling, for example a brother or sister who is himself/herself a psychiatrist or psychologist, or has a prestige of one kind or another in his family, is the one who encourages family therapy, then be careful about making it, because this very sibling can be at the root of the family pathology. These are not only recurring clues for us, but for other therapists too.[1] If they heed it and it proves true, they have the means of doing good therapy. And that's why we are not interested in inventing stories.

WEBER: What you say makes quite clear why Carl Auer is a suspect figure for you.

MARA SELVINI PALAZZOLI: Carl Auer a suspect? No! In my opinion he represents a particular line of thinking that I no longer share.

MATTEO SELVINI: He represents this radical constructivism. . . .

MARA SELVINI PALAZZOLI: . . . which in itself is a very positive thing: it's the botch-up some family therapists have made of it that it is so detrimental. They have often used it for therapeutical relativism and nihilism.

MATTEO SELVINI: . . . and to free themselves from therapeutical responsibility.

WEBER: We thank you for this interview.

[1] Selvini Palazzoli, M.: "The problem of the sibling as the referring person," *Journal of Marital and Family Therapy*, 11, 21-34, 1985.

Epilogue
Targets on the Truth - Annotated Chronological Table

Do we not frequently experience that wild fantasies prove to be well-founded, and what seem to be facts turn out to be falsities?

In reference to an exact inquiry into the life and work of Carl Auer this volume can only be the starting point for a careful search for tracks. And yet it provides us with a great number of surprising clues and details. Since all the contributors to this acknowledgment and collection of information are scientists, doctors and psycho-therapists of some reputation, their reports can be considered largely as reliable documents and historical sources. In order to present a first rough summary of Carl Auer´s journey through life we have tried to extract all the important "hard" information from the dense personal accounts of the various authors, put them together in the form of a table and to comment on them. Where we were in possession of material that is not directly referred to in this book (e.g. film material), we have also integrated this knowledge in the chronological table.

1900 Up till now we have practically no reliable information about his early childhood and his parental home. Only one thing seems to be clear: he was born in a small village on the Swiss south bank of Lake Constance, which has meanwhile been incorporated into the climatic health resort of Rorschach, and grew up in the second district of Vienna, where Sigmund Freud lived with his family, too. It has been hinted that he is the illegitimate child of an Italian opera singer. Bertha, one of his father's sisters who lived nearby, was the person to whom he related most closely. He had contacts with the Freud family through friendship with Freud's niece Annabella. Over and above this there are indications that relations existed between the Auer family and the Einsteins. The assumptions that Carl Auer is Albert Einstein's first cousin could not be verified to this day. However, Auer's second wife, Jelena, had an intensive interchange with Einstein's wife Milena later.

1910   Started at the same grammar school which Heinz von Foerster was to attend later.

1914   Important personal insights (content unknown, but probably connected with the outbreak of the First World War).

1917   Passed his 'A' levels with mediocre results.

1918   Participation in the First World War (on the Austrian side). Wounded and made prisoner of war in Italy. In captivity he was cell mate to Ludwig Wittgenstein in Monte Cassino.

1922-23 Student and at the same time private tutor; gave the young Heinz von Foerster private tuition in mathematics, for example.

1924   Marriage to E. Wald. First emigration to the United States of America (Wisconsin). His marriage to E. Wald produced the sons Edgar and Normal Auerswald.

1926-27 Sojourn in Chile. Acquaintance with mother of Maturana.

1927-29 Studied art in Paris (with Fernand Léger among others). Acquaintance with mother of Hoffman at an opening day of the sculptor Ossip Zadkine.

1929-34	Achieved temporary fame under the name of Leonard Zelig first in the United States, then in Europe.
1934	Return to Vienna, studied psychoanalysis.
1936	Teaching post at the University of Vienna (probably chemistry, at all events continued analytical work). What contact he had to Ludwig von Bertalanffy, who taught biology there at that time, remains obscure.
1936	Separation from E. Wald.
1937-38	Psychoanalysis in the United States.
1938	Operation in Mexico City (sex change?).
1938	Encounter with Ernst von Glasersfeld on a glacier in the Austrian Alps. At this time occupation as editor of left-wing newspaper in Vienna. First acquaintance with his second wife-to-be, Jelena Kuss. This marriage produced two children, Carl-Anton and Nina. After Anschluß of Austria to the German Reich he fled to Switzerland.
1939	Honorary citizen of Appenzell ("Rescuer of Appenzell").
1940-45	Visiting professor at University of Canterbury/New Zealand. Begin of long friendship with Karl Popper.
1942	Vacation in U.S.A. Stayed with Peggy Penn's family in the Penn(!)sylvanian Hills.
1945	Return to Europe. For the first months stayed with the Enderlin family in Switzerland.
1946-47	Teaching post at the Swiss Technical College in Zurich. Then began a time of intensive travel.

1948	Was occupied for several months in the Chestnut Lodge Sanitarium near Washington D.C.
1949	Met André Gide in Paris (there is no proof of a suspected homosexual relationship). Afterwards journey to Haiti where he called himself Charles d'Auer and cultivated intensive contacts with Voodoo priests.
1950	Stayed in Italy. Ernst von Glasersfeld listened to one of his lectures there. In Heidelberg he then held his meanwhile famous Heidelberg lectures. Towards the end of the year Helm Stierlin thinks he met him in the Black Forest, where Auer had gone for a rest. An encounter with Heidegger is probable. We know for certain that the insight that "nothingness is of itself none" was originally Auer's. The second half of this profound piece of writing "... and the hole is essentially hole-istic" was not adopted by Heidegger as an integral part of his philosophy.
1951	Return to the U.S.A. In Phoenix, Arizona he met Milton Erickson, of almost the same age, and Jack Daniels, who was twelve at the time. He left practically no tracks for almost two decades, the few facts and clues available are not sufficiently substantiated.
1959	Practiced psychotherapy in Vienna (?)
1969	Separation from wife Jelena.
1976 - 77	Stayed in Milwaukee where a street was named after him.
1978 - 80	Planned a "new town" in Arcosanti in the Arizona desert together with Paolo Soleri and a young Mexican architect.

1980 - 85   Work on chaos theory.

1985   Travelled to Australia and New Zealand to his former place of work. Encountered David Epston.

1985 - 88   Head of the United Nations World Coincidence Control Center (Wocococ).

1988   Journey to Europe. Hiking in the Odenwald near Heidelberg. Meeting with A. Retzer, F.B. Simon and G. Weber on 22nd November, agreement on the arrangements for publishing a *festschrift* in his honour and on setting up a publishing house.

1988 - 90   For the past two years Auer has lived a secluded life on Coney Island as silent partner of an amusement park.